DIABETES GASTROPARESIS DIET COOKBOOK

Doctor-Approved Delicious Recipes and Strategies for Living Well with Gastroparesis and Diabetes | with 30 Days Meal Plan

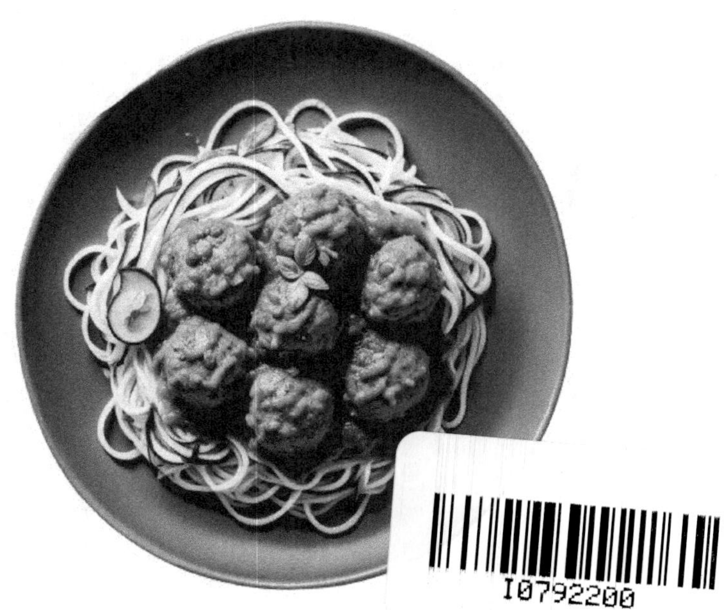

Dr. Alma W. Thygesen

Disclaimer:

The information contained in this book is for informational purposes only an' is not a substitute for professional medical advice. Always consult with a qualified healthcare professional before makin' any changes to your diet or exercise routine.

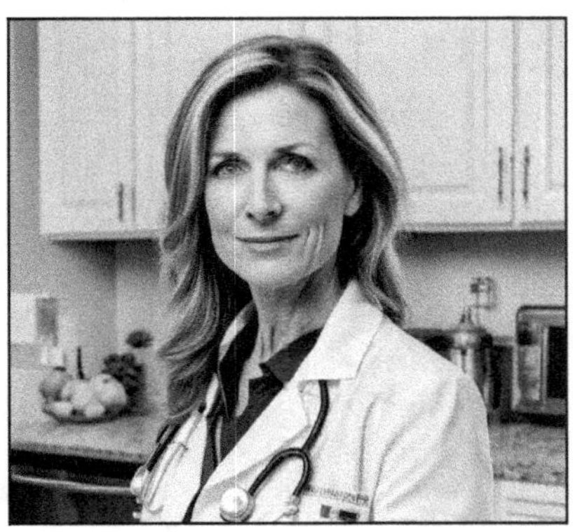

<u>Dr. Alma W. Thygesen</u>

I am Dr. Alma W. Thygesen, your go to doc, researcher, an' health enthusiast, balancin' life between Malibu's sunshine an' the hustle of being a wife an' mom. You can find me at Seaside Medical Center, nestled in the heart of Malibu, where I am dedicated to providin' exceptional care to all who come my way. When I am not in the clinic, you'll find me enjoyin' the coastal breeze, embracin' the Malibu lifestyle, an' cherishin' moments with my wonderful family.

My journey in medicine began at UCLA, where my passion for healin' blossomed. Later, I ventured to Stanford University for specialized trainin', honin' my skills to better serve my community. Now, I merge cuttin' edge research with heartfelt empathy, ensurin' every individual's well being, one patient at a time.

<u>Preface: The Untold Story of Sarah an' Gastroparesis</u>

For years, Sarah knew somethin' wasn't right. A naggin' feelin' of fullness after meals, a constant battle with nausea, an' an inexplicable weight loss became her unwelcome companions. Visitin' doctor after doctor, she searched for answers, only to be met with a confusin' maze of tests an' inconclusive results. Finally, a diagnosis arrived – gastroparesis. Relief washed over her, not because the condition was easy, but because she finally had a name for the struggle she'd endured for so long.

Gastroparesis, a debilitatin' digestive disorder that weakens the stomach muscles, became Sarah's unwelcome teacher. It forced her to confront her limitations, to mourn the spontaneous meals an' social gatherings that once brought her joy. Simple tasks like grocery shoppin' an' meal preppin' transformed into intricate calculations, balancin' nutritional needs with what her stomach could tolerate.

Yet, Sarah was a fighter. She refused to let gastroparesis define her. With unwaverin' determination, she embarked on a journey of self discovery. She devoured research on the condition, connectin' with online communities an' learnin' from others' experiences. She partnered with a registered dietitian, craftin' a meal plan that nourished her body without triggerin' her symptoms. Mindful of the mind body connection, she incorporated stress management techniques, findin' solace in yoga an' meditation.

This book is a testament to Sarah's resilience. It's a culmination of her experiences, a roadmap for others grapplin' with the complexities of gastroparesis an' diabetes. Within these pages, you'll find not only practical guidance on managin' these conditions but also a profound message of hope. Sarah's story reminds us that even in the face of adversity, we can find strength, creativity, an' the power to reclaim control of our well being.

So, whether you're newly diagnosed or a seasoned warrior in the fight against gastroparesis an' diabetes, know this: you are not alone. This book is here to guide you, to empower you, an' to inspire you on your own journey towards a healthier, happier you.

Table of contents

Part 1: Understanding Diabetes and Gastroparesis

Chapter 1: Introduction

Livin' with a Double Diagnosis

Havin' diabetes an' gastroparesis simultaneously can feel like navigatin' a tightrope. You're managin' two complex conditions, each with its own set of challenges. Diabetes disrupts your body's ability to regulate blood sugar, while gastroparesis throws a wrench in your digestive system. It's a balancin' act, but with the right approach, you can find a path to feelin' better.

The Frustration Factor:

One of the biggest hurdles can be the frustration of seemingly contradictory needs. For example, diabetes often requires eatin' regular meals to maintain blood sugar levels. But gastroparesis might make frequent, larger meals difficult to digest. This can lead to discouragement an' a feelin' of being trapped.

Understandin' the Link:

The good news is that there's a connection between the two. Uncontrolled blood sugar can actually worsen gastroparesis symptoms. So, by managin' your diabetes effectively, you're indirectly helpin' your digestive system. This can be a powerful motivator to stay on top of your blood sugar control.

Findin' the Right Support:

Livin' with a double diagnosis requires a strong support system. This can include a healthcare team that understands both conditions an' can create a personalized treatment plan. A registered dietitian can be a lifesaver, helpin' you craft a diet that addresses both your blood sugar an' your digestion needs. Don't hesitate to reach out to support groups or communities where you can connect with others who understand your struggles.

The Importance of Diet Management

Diet management plays a critical role in navigatin' the challenges of both diabetes an' gastroparesis. Here's why it is so important:

Blood Sugar Control:

- **Diabetes:** In diabetes, your body struggles to regulate blood sugar levels. The right diet helps manage this by:

    - **Fiber**: Includin' soluble fiber slows down carbohydrate absorption, preventin' blood sugar spikes.

    - **Portion Control**: Eatin' smaller, more frequent meals prevents overwhelmin' your system an' causin' sugar surges.

    - **Food Choices**: Selectin' low glycemic index foods minimizes rapid blood sugar rise.

Gastroparesis Relief:

- **Gastroparesis**: This condition slows down stomach emptyin', leadin' to discomfort. Diet management helps by:

    - **Smaller Meals**: Eatin' smaller portions frequently eases digestion an' reduces nausea, bloatin', an' vomitin'.

    - **Liquid Intake**: Consumin' liquids like broths an' smoothies ensures proper hydration an' provides nutrients easier on the stomach.

    - **Low Fiber Options**: Limitin' high fiber foods that can be difficult to digest improves food movement through the stomach.

<u>**A Synergistic Approach:**</u>

The beauty lies in the synergy between these benefits. By managin' your diabetes with diet, you can indirectly help your gastroparesis. For example, better blood sugar control can improve nerve function in your stomach, leadin' to more efficient digestion.

<u>**A Personalized Plan:**</u>

There's no one size fits all approach. A registered dietitian can create a personalized plan considerin' your:

- **Blood Sugar Levels**: Tailorin' carbohydrate intake to manage your diabetes.

- **Gastroparesis Symptoms**: Identifyin' foods you tolerate best to minimize discomfort.

- **Nutritional Needs**: Ensurin' you receive all essential vitamins an' minerals for optimal health.

<u>**Takin' Charge of Your Wellbeing:**</u>

By prioritizin' diet management, you become an active participant in managin' both diabetes an' gastroparesis. This empowers you to:

- **Reduce Symptoms**: Experience fewer gastroparesis flare ups an' improve blood sugar control.

- **Improve Quality of Life**: Enjoy a more active an' fulfillin' life with less discomfort.

- **Prevent Complications**: Minimize the risk of long term complications associated with both conditions.

Chapter 2: Demystifying Diabetes: Types, Causes, and Management Strategies

Unveilin' the Different Forms of Diabetes

Diabetes might seem like a single condition, but it actually encompasses several variations, each with its own cause an' characteristics. Below is an explanation of the most prevalent types:

1. Type 1 Diabetes:

- ★ **The Autoimmune Culprit**: This type arises when your body's immune system mistakenly attacks the insulin producin' cells in your pancreas.

- ★ **Lifelong Dependence**: As a result, your body produces little to no insulin, necessitatin' lifelong insulin injections to manage blood sugar levels.

- ★ **Onset**: Often diagnosed in childhood or young adulthood.

2. Type 2 Diabetes:

- **Insulin Resistance**: This is the most common form of diabetes. Your body still produces insulin, but it becomes resistant to its effects, leadin' to high blood sugar levels.

- **Lifestyle Factors**: Risk factors include genetics, weight, physical inactivity, an' unhealthy diet.

- **Management Strategies**: Treatment may involve lifestyle changes like diet an' exercise, oral medications, or injectable medications.

3. <u>Gestational Diabetes:</u>

- **Pregnancy Related**: This form develops durin' pregnancy due to hormonal changes that can affect insulin sensitivity.

- **Temporary**: It usually resolves after childbirth, but women with gestational diabetes have a higher risk of developin' type 2 diabetes later in life.

- **Management Focuses on:** Maintainin' healthy blood sugar levels for the well being of both mother an' baby.

<u>Beyond the Big Three:</u>

While less common, other types of diabetes exist, such as:

- **Maturity onset diabetes of the young (MODY)**: A genetic form of diabetes with various subtypes.

- **Neonatal diabetes**: A rare form diagnosed in infancy.

- **Secondary diabetes**: Caused by other medical conditions or medications.

<u>Understandin' Your Type:</u>

Knowin' your specific type of diabetes is crucial. It helps your doctor create a personalized treatment plan that addresses the root cause an' effectively manages your blood sugar levels. Tests like blood sugar level checks an' antibody tests can help determine your type.

The Takeaway:

Diabetes may have different faces, but its core issue high blood sugar remains the same.

Understandin' How Diabetes Affects Your Body

Diabetes throws a wrench into the delicate dance of how your body processes food an' maintains energy levels. Here's a breakdown of how it disrupts this symphony:

The Role of Insulin:

Imagine insulin as a key. It unlocks the doors of your cells, allowin' sugar (glucose) from your bloodstream to enter an' be used for energy.

The Diabetic Disruption:

- **Type 1 Diabetes**: In this case, the key maker (pancreas) is malfunctionin', producin' little to no insulin.

- **Type 2 Diabetes**: Here, the cells become resistant to the key (insulin), makin' it harder for sugar to enter.

Consequences of High Blood Sugar:

With the "doors" locked, sugar builds up in the bloodstream, leadin' to:

- **Cellular Starvation**: Cells become starved for energy despite the presence of sugar in the bloodstream.

- **Increased Thirst an' Urination**: The body tries to expel excess sugar through urine, leadin' to dehydration an' frequent urination.

- **Long Term Complications**: Over time, chronically high blood sugar can damage nerves, blood vessels, an' organs, increasin' the risk of heart disease, stroke, kidney disease, an' vision problems.

The Body's Response:

- **The Pancreas (Type 2):** In type 2 diabetes, the pancreas may try to compensate by producin' more insulin, but eventually may struggle to keep up.

- **The Liver:** The liver tries to help by producin' some glucose, further contributin' to high blood sugar levels.

<u>A Domino Effect:</u>

Uncontrolled diabetes can trigger a domino effect, with high blood sugar damagin' blood vessels an' nerves throughout the body. This can lead to a cascade of health problems if not managed effectively.

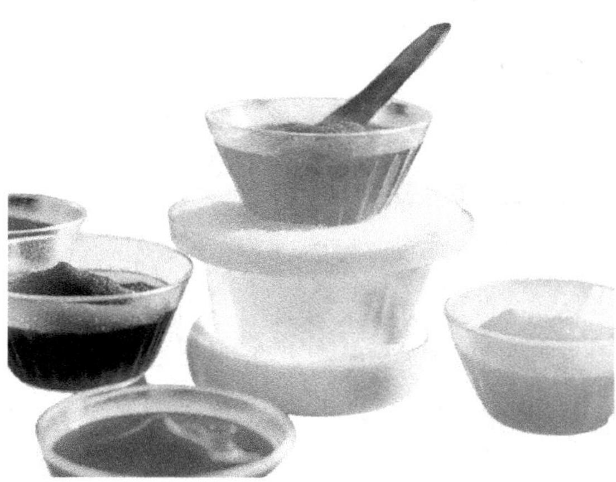

Blood Sugar Control: Your Key to Well being

Blood sugar control is the cornerstone of managin' diabetes, an' for good reason. It's like the master switch that regulates your body's energy flow an' overall well being. Here's why keepin' your blood sugar in check is crucial:

Maintainin' Cellular Harmony:

Imagine your body's cells as tiny factories. They need a steady supply of sugar (glucose) for fuel to function properly. When blood sugar levels are within a healthy range, insulin acts as a key, unlockin' the cell doors an' allowin' sugar to enter for energy production.

The Domino Effect of Uncontrolled Blood Sugar:

If blood sugar levels become chronically high (hyperglycemia), a domino effect unfolds:

- **Cellular Starvation**: Cells become locked out from their fuel source, leadin' to fatigue an' other health issues.

- **Organ Damage**: Over time, high blood sugar can damage nerves, blood vessels, an' organs, increasin' the risk of heart disease, stroke, kidney disease, an' vision problems.

The Benefits of Balanced Blood Sugar:

By keepin' your blood sugar levels within a healthy range, you unlock a treasure chest of benefits:

- **Improved Energy Levels**: With a steady supply of fuel to your cells, you'll experience increased energy an' vitality.

- **Reduced Risk of Complications**: You significantly decrease your risk of developin' serious diabetes related health problems.

- **Enhanced Quality of Life**: Effective blood sugar control allows you to live a more active an' fulfillin' life.

Takin' Charge of Your Blood Sugar:

The good news is that you have the power to influence your blood sugar levels through several key strategies:

- **Healthy Diet**: Choose a balanced diet rich in complex carbohydrates, fiber, an' lean proteins to regulate sugar absorption.

- **Regular Exercise**: Physical activity helps your body use sugar for energy, naturally lowerin' blood sugar levels.

- **Weight Management**: Maintainin' a healthy weight reduces insulin resistance, makin' it easier for your body to utilize sugar.

- **Medication (if needed):** In some cases, medications like insulin may be necessary to manage blood sugar effectively.

Blood Sugar Monitorin':

Regular blood sugar monitorin' is essential. It allows you to track your progress, identify patterns, an' adjust your management strategies as needed. Workin' alongside your doctor, you can establish a personalized blood sugar monitorin' plan.

Blood Sugar Control: Your Investment in Health:

Blood sugar control is an investment in your long term health an' well being. By prioritizin' it, you're takin' an active role in managin' your diabetes an' pavin' the way for a healthier, more vibrant future.

Chapter 3: Gastroparesis Explained: Causes

What is Gastroparesis an' Why Does it Happen?

The human digestive system is a complex orchestra, with each organ playin' a crucial role in breakin' down food an' absorbin' nutrients. In gastroparesis, this harmony is disrupted, leadin' to a frustratin' an' often debilitatin' condition. Let's delve into the world of gastroparesis, understandin' what it is an' the reasons behind this digestive slowdown.

The Stomach's Role:

Imagine the stomach as a muscular sac that acts as a temporary holdin' station for food. Its powerful muscles churn an' break down ingested food into a liquid mixture called chyme. This chyme is then slowly released into the small intestine for further digestion an' nutrient absorption.

The Gastroparesis Disruption:

In gastroparesis, the normal muscular contractions of the stomach weaken or become delayed. This disrupts the stomach's ability to efficiently process an' empty food. As a result, food sits in the stomach for extended periods, leadin' to a cascade of problems.

Causes of the Disruption:

The exact reasons behind gastroparesis remain under investigation. However, several factors are known to contribute:

- **Nerve Damage:** Damage to the vagus nerve, which controls stomach muscle contractions, can be a culprit. This damage might be caused by diabetes (a common association), viral infections, or surgical procedures.

- **Autoimmune Disorders**: In some cases, the immune system mistakenly attacks healthy stomach muscles, weakenin' their function.

- **Idiopathic Gastroparesis**: In many instances, no clear cause is identified. This form is known as idiopathic gastroparesis.

The Domino Effect of Delayed Gastric Emptyin':

Food sittin' for too long in the stomach can lead to a domino effect:

- **Bacterial Overgrowth**: Bacteria present in the stomach can multiply excessively, contributin' to bloatin' an' nausea.

- **Incomplete Digestion**: Nutrients from the food may not be properly absorbed, leadin' to malnutrition an' deficiencies.

- **Gastroparesis Symptoms**: Symptoms like nausea, vomitin', abdominal pain, early satiety (feelin' full after eatin' a small amount), an' heartburn become a constant struggle.

Understandin' Gastroparesis is Key:

Gastroparesis, while challengin', is not a life sentence. By understandin' the underlyin' causes an' workin' with your doctor, you can develop a personalized management plan to alleviate symptoms an' improve your quality of life.

Recognizin' the Signs an' Symptoms

Gastroparesis, often referred to as "stomach paralysis," disrupts the normal rhythm of your digestive system. This can lead to a range of uncomfortable symptoms that can significantly impact your daily life. Here's a breakdown of the key signs an' symptoms to watch out for:

Upper Gastrointestinal Discomfort:

- **Nausea an' Vomitin'**: These are hallmark symptoms of gastroparesis. You might experience frequent nausea, or even forceful vomitin' of undigested food.

- **Abdominal Pain an' Discomfort**: A persistent dull ache or gnawin' pain in the upper abdomen can be a sign that your stomach is strugglin' to empty its contents.

- **Bloatin' an' Feelin' Full**: Even after eatin' a small amount, you might feel uncomfortably full an' bloated due to food lin'erin' in your stomach.

- **Loss of Appetite**: The constant discomfort an' nausea can lead to a decreased appetite, makin' it difficult to maintain proper nutrition.

Digestive Issues:

- **Early Satiety**: The feelin' of fullness after just a few bites is a telltale sign of gastroparesis. Your stomach fills up quickly, leavin' no room for a complete meal.

- **Heartburn an' Acid Reflux**: Delayed stomach emptyin' can cause stomach acid to back up into the esophagus, leadin' to heartburn an' a burnin' sensation in the chest.

- **Weight Loss:** Due to difficulty eatin' an' malabsorption of nutrients, unintended weight loss can be a common consequence of gastroparesis.

<u>**Beyond the Digestive Tract:**</u>

- **Fatigue an' Weakness**: The body's struggle to absorb nutrients can lead to fatigue an' a general lack of energy.

- **Dehydration**: Gastroparesis may cause difficulty keepin' fluids down, leadin' to dehydration an' its associated symptoms like dizziness an' headaches.

- **Nutritional Deficiencies**: Long term malabsorption of nutrients can lead to deficiencies in vitamins an' minerals, impactin' overall health.

<u>**Not Every Symptom Spells Gastroparesis:**</u>

It's important to note that these symptoms can also be associated with other digestive conditions. If you experience any of these signs persistently, consult your doctor for a proper diagnosis. Early diagnosis an' management are crucial for controllin' symptoms an' improvin' your quality of life.

<u>**Listen to Your Body:**</u>

By becomin' familiar with the signs an' symptoms of gastroparesis, you can be more attuned to your body's signals. This empowers you to discuss your concerns with your doctor an' work towards a solution for a healthier digestive future.

Explorin' Treatment Approaches for Relief

Livin' with gastroparesis can be frustratin', but there are treatment options available to help manage symptoms an' improve your quality of life. Let's delve into the various approaches you can explore with your doctor:

Dietary Modifications:

- **Smaller, More Frequent Meals**: Eatin' smaller portions throughout the day puts less stress on your stomach, promotin' easier digestion.

- **Focus on Liquids**: Liquids an' soft foods are easier to digest than solid foods. Smoothies, soups, an' pureed vegetables can be good options.

- **Low Fiber Diet**: Fiber can be difficult to digest for some with gastroparesis. Limitin' high fiber foods like whole grains an' raw vegetables may be necessary.

- **Hydration is Key**: Drinkin' plenty of fluids throughout the day helps to prevent dehydration, a common concern in gastroparesis. Electrolyte rich beverages can be particularly beneficial.

Medications:

- **Prokinetics**: These medications stimulate the muscles in your stomach to help it empty more efficiently. Examples include metoclopramide an' erythromycin.

- **Anti Nausea Medication**: Medications like ondansetron or promethazine can help control nausea an' vomitin', easin' discomfort.

- **Pain Management**: Medications may be prescribed to manage abdominal pain associated with gastroparesis.

<u>**Nutritional Support:**</u>

- **Nutritional Supplements**: If dietary intake is insufficient, your doctor may recommend oral nutritional supplements or even intravenous feedin' to ensure you receive the essential nutrients your body needs.

<u>**Interventional Procedures:**</u>

- **Gastric Feedin' Tube**: In severe cases, a feedin' tube placed directly into the small intestine can bypass the stomach an' deliver liquid nutrition.

- **Endoscopic Botulinum Toxin Injection (BTX):** This minimally invasive procedure injects Botox into the pyloric sphincter (muscle at the stomach exit) to relax it an' improve stomach emptyin'.

- **Gastric Peroral Endoscopic Myotomy (G-POEM):** This newer endoscopic procedure creates a small incision in the pyloric sphincter to facilitate smoother stomach emptyin'.

<u>**Stress Management Techniques:**</u>

Chronic stress can worsen gastroparesis symptoms. Techniques like yoga, meditation, an' relaxation exercises can be helpful in managin' stress an' potentially improvin' your digestive well being.

Chapter 4: Dietary Guidelines for Success: Balancing Blood Sugar and Digestion

Prioritizin' Nutrient Intake for Optimal Health

Livin' with both diabetes an' gastroparesis presents a unique challenge: balancin' blood sugar control with the need for easily digestible foods. But fear not! By prioritizin' nutrient intake, you can ensure your body receives the essential buildin' blocks for optimal health. Here's how:

Understandin' Your Needs:

- **Macronutrients**: Focus on a balanced intake of macronutrients – carbohydrates, protein, an' healthy fats.

- **Carbohydrates**: Choose complex carbohydrates like vegetables an' some fruits for sustained energy without blood sugar spikes.

- **Protein**: Include lean protein sources like fish, poultry, an' legumes for muscle buildin', satiety, an' blood sugar control.

- **Healthy Fats**: Don't shy away from healthy fats like avocado, nuts, an' olive oil. They provide satiety, aid vitamin absorption, an' support overall health.

- **Micronutrients**: Don't forget the power of micronutrients – vitamins an' minerals. They play crucial roles in various bodily functions an' can be impacted by gastroparesis.

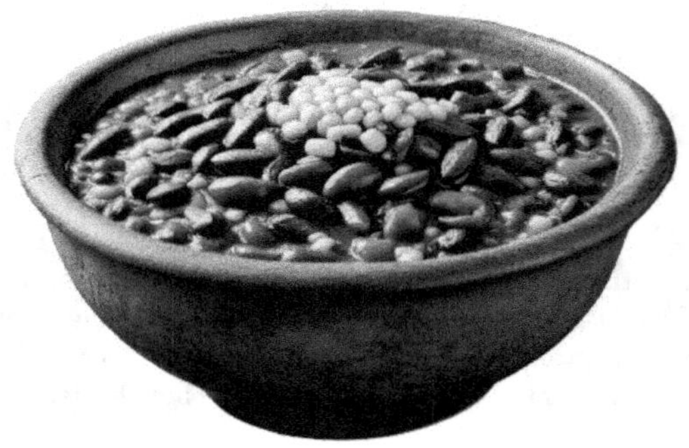

Makin' Smart Food Choices:

- **Focus on Nutrient Density**: Choose nutrient dense foods that pack a punch of vitamins an' minerals in every bite. Examples include leafy green vegetables, berries, an' lean protein sources.

- **Liquids an' Soft Foods**: Since some solid foods might be difficult to digest, incorporate liquids like smoothies an' soups. You can also include soft, cooked vegetables an' mashed potatoes.

- **Low Fiber Options**: While fiber is generally beneficial, it can be challengin' to digest for some with gastroparesis. Opt for low fiber options like peeled fruits an' refined grains until your tolerance improves.

Addressin' Potential Deficiencies:

- **Nutritional Supplements**: If dietary intake is insufficient due to gastroparesis limitations, your doctor may recommend oral nutritional supplements. These can bridge the gap an' ensure you receive essential vitamins an' minerals.

Choosin' the Right Foods for Gastroparesis Tolerance

Gastroparesis throws a curveball at your digestive system, makin' it challengin' to find foods that go down smoothly. But fret not! By understandin' which foods are easier to digest an' incorporatin' them into your diet, you can navigate mealtimes with more comfort. Here's a breakdown of food choices that can be your gastroparesis friendly allies:

Liquids an' Soft Foods: Your Digestive BFFs

- **Smoothies**: Blend fruits, vegetables, yogurt, or protein powder for a nutrient packed an' easily digestible drink.

- **Soups**: Broth based soups with cooked, softened vegetables are gentle on your stomach an' keep you hydrated.

- **Applesauce an' Mashed Fruits**: These provide sweetness an' essential vitamins in a form that's easy on your digestive system.

- **Yogurt (plain or Greek):** A good source of protein an' probiotics, which can aid digestion. Choose low fat options an' limit added sugars.

- **Well Cooked Vegetables**: Cookin' vegetables breaks down their fiber content, makin' them easier to digest. Steamin', roastin', or boilin' are good options.

- **Mashed Potatoes**: Mashed potatoes offer a source of complex carbohydrates for sustained energy without being overly taxin' on your stomach.

Solid Foods to Consider (Introduce Gradually):

- **White Rice an' Refined Grains**: These are easier to digest than whole grains due to their lower fiber content. Introduce them gradually an' in moderation.

- **Skinless, Cooked Chicken or Fish**: Lean protein sources are essential for buildin' an' maintainin' muscle mass. Opt for well cooked options for easier digestion.

- **Eggs**: Eggs are a complete protein source, providin' all the essential amino acids your body needs. Scrambled or soft boiled eggs are gentler on the stomach.

- **Ripe Fruits**: Bananas, melons, an' other ripe fruits are generally well tolerated due to their soft texture an' easily absorbed sugars.

Foods to Limit or Avoid:

- **High Fiber Foods**: Raw vegetables, whole grains, nuts, an' seeds can be difficult to digest due to their high fiber content.

- **Fatty or Fried Foods**: These foods take longer to digest an' can irritate your stomach.

- **Spicy Foods**: Spicy foods can trigger heartburn an' discomfort in some individuals with gastroparesis.

- **Carbonated Drinks**: The fizz in carbonated drinks can cause bloatin' an' discomfort. Opt for water or clear broths instead.

- **Alcohol**: Alcohol can slow down stomach emptyin' an' worsen gastroparesis symptoms.

Remember:

Individual Tolerance: Every person with gastroparesis has different tolerance levels. Experiment gradually to see what works best for you.

Managin' Blood Sugar Levels with Smart Meal Plannin'

For people with diabetes, managin' blood sugar levels is crucial for maintainin' overall health. Smart meal plannin' empowers you to take control of your diet an' achieve optimal blood sugar control. Here's how to become a meal plannin' maestro for your diabetic well being:

The Power of Plate Proportion:

Imagine your plate as a canvas for a balanced masterpiece. Here's how to strategically fill it:

- **Half the Plate**: Non starchy vegetables like leafy greens, broccoli, or peppers take center stage. They're low in calories an' carbohydrates, providin' essential vitamins an' fiber without spikin' blood sugar.

- **Quarter of the Plate**: Lean protein sources like grilled chicken, fish, or beans come next. Protein helps with satiety an' can contribute to steadier blood sugar levels.

- **Quarter of the Plate**: This is your dedicated carbohydrate zone. Choose whole grains like brown rice or quinoa, starchy vegetables like sweet potatoes, or fruits like berries. Opt for whole grains over refined options for sustained energy an' a lower glycemic index impact.

Portion Control is Key:

Even healthy foods can affect blood sugar if eaten in excess. Use measurin' cups or bowls to ensure you're servin' yourself appropriate portions.

Spreadin' the Wealth:

Don't cram all your carbohydrates into one meal. Distribute them throughout the day to avoid blood sugar spikes. Aim for 3 balanced meals an' 2 - 3 healthy snacks.

Fiber is Your Friend:

Fiber slows down the absorption of sugar into your bloodstream, preventin' blood sugar spikes. Include plenty of fiber rich options like vegetables, fruits, an' whole grains in your meals an' snacks.

Readin' Food Labels:

Food labels are your allies. Pay attention to servin' sizes, carbohydrate content, an' sugar content. This knowledge empowers you to make informed choices that align with your blood sugar management goals.

Plannin' Makes Perfect:

Takin' an hour each week to plan your meals an' snacks sets you up for success. This way, you'll have healthy options readily available an' avoid unhealthy choices when hunger strikes.

Beyond the Plate:

Remember, meal plannin' is just one piece of the puzzle. Regular exercise, managin' stress, an' gettin' enough sleep all contribute to better blood sugar control.

Embrace Variety:

A balanced an' varied diet keeps things interestin' an' ensures you're gettin' a full spectrum of nutrients. Explore new recipes an' healthy ingredients to keep your taste buds happy.

With smart meal plannin', you can transform mealtimes from a source of stress to an empowerin' act of self care for your diabetic health.

Recipes

Breakfast

Scrambled Eggs with Spinach an' Goat Cheese

Prep Time: 15 minutes

Ingredients:
- 4 eggs
- 1 cup fresh spinach
- 1/4 cup crumbled goat cheese
- Salt an' pepper to taste

Step by step instructions:
1. Whisk eggs in a bowl an' season with salt an' pepper.
2. Heat a skillet over medium heat an' add spinach, cookin' until wilted.
3. Pour in the whisked eggs an' cook, stirrin' occasionally, until nearly set.
4. Sprinkle crumbled goat cheese over the eggs an' continue cookin' until melted.
5. Serve hot.

Nutritional data (approximate) for each servin':
- Calories: 280
- Protein: 19g
- Carbohydrates: 3g
- Fat: 21g

Suggestions for freezin' an' storage:
- Store any leftovers in an airtight container in the refrigerator for up to 2 days. Reheat gently in the microwave.

Reasons why this recipe stands out:
- Offers a flavorful twist on traditional scrambled eggs with the addition of creamy goat cheese an' nutritious spinach.

Protein Smoothie with Berries an' Unsweetened Greek Yogurt

Prep Time: 5 minutes

Ingredients:

- 1 cup mixed berries (strawberries, blueberries, raspberries)
- 1/2 cup unsweetened Greek yogurt
- 1 scoop protein powder (flavor of your choice)
- 1/2 cup water or almond milk

Step by step instructions:
1. Combine all ingredients in a blender.
2. Blend until smooth an' creamy.
3. Add more liquid if needed to reach desired consistency.
4. Pour into a glass an' enjoy immediately.

Nutritional data (approximate) for each servin':
- Calories: 250
- Protein: 25g
- Carbohydrates: 20g
- Fat: 8g

Suggestions for freezin' an' storage:
- Smoothies are best enjoyed fresh but can be stored in the refrigerator for up to 24 hours.

Reasons why this recipe stands out:
- Packs a powerful protein punch while providin' a refreshin' an' delicious way to start your day.

Chia Seed Puddin' with Nut Butter an' Sliced Strawberries

Prep Time: 5 minutes (+overnight chillin')

Ingredients:

- 1/4 cup chia seeds
- 1 cup almond milk
- 1 tablespoon nut butter (almond, peanut, or cashew)
- Sliced strawberries for toppin'

Step by step instructions:
1. In a jar or bowl, mix chia seeds an' almond milk.
2. Add nut butter an' stir well to combine.
3. Cover an' refrigerate overnight or for at least 4 hours until thickened.
4. Serve topped with sliced strawberries.

Nutritional data (approximate) for each servin':
- Calories: 220
- Protein: 7g
- Carbohydrates: 18g
- Fat: 14g

Suggestions for freezin' an' storage:
- Chia seed puddin' can be stored in the refrigerator for up to 3 days. Stir well before servin'.

Reasons why this recipe stands out:
- Offers a nutritious an' satisfyin' breakfast option that's rich in omega 3 fatty acids an' protein, with a delicious nutty flavor.

Baked Oatmeal with Apples an' Cinnamon (use sugar substitutes like stevia)

Prep Time: 10 minutes

Ingredients:

- 2 cups rolled oats
- 2 cups unsweetened almond milk
- 2 apples, diced
- 2 teaspoons cinnamon
- Stevia or other sugar substitutes to taste

Step by step instructions:
1. Preheat oven to 350°F (175°C).
2. In a mixin' bowl, combine oats, almond milk, diced apples, cinnamon, an' sugar substitute.
3. Pour mixture into a greased bakin' dish.
4. Bake for 30 35 minutes or until golden an' set.
5. Serve warm.

Nutritional data (approximate) for each servin':
- Calories: 220
- Protein: 6g
- Carbohydrates: 40g
- Fat: 4g

Suggestions for freezin' an' storage:
- Allow baked oatmeal to cool completely, then store in an airtight container in the refrigerator for up to 5 days. Reheat gently in the microwave.

Reasons why this recipe stands out:
- Provides a comfortin' an' nutritious breakfast option with the natural sweetness of apples an' warm cinnamon flavor, without added sugars.

Cottage Cheese Pancakes with Berries (use sugar free pancake mix)

Prep Time: 15 minutes

Ingredients:

- Sugar free pancake mix
- Water or milk (accordin' to pancake mix instructions)
- Cottage cheese
- Mixed berries for toppin'

Step by step instructions:
1. Prepare pancake batter accordin' to package instructions, substitutin' water or milk for a liquid component if needed.
2. Fold in cottage cheese into the batter.
3. Heat a non stick skillet over medium heat an' pour batter to form pancakes.
4. Cook until bubbles appear, then flip an' cook the other side until golden brown.
5. Serve hot with mixed berries on top.

Nutritional data (approximate) for each servin':
- Calories: 200
- Protein: 10g
- Carbohydrates: 30g
- Fat: 5g

Suggestions for freezin' an' storage:
- Freeze pancakes individually on a bakin' sheet, then transfer to a freezer bag for up to 3 months. Thaw an' reheat in the toaster or microwave.

Reasons why this recipe stands out:
- Incorporates cottage cheese for added protein an' a fluffy texture, while usin' sugar free pancake mix for a healthier twist.

Egg Muffins with Vegetables an' Ham

Prep Time: 20 minutes

Ingredients:
- 6 eggs
- 1/2 cup diced ham
- 1/2 cup diced vegetables (bell peppers, onions, spinach, etc.)
- Salt an' pepper to taste

Step by step instructions:
1. Preheat oven to 350°F (175°C) an' grease a muffin tin.
2. In a bowl, whisk together eggs, salt, an' pepper.
3. Stir in diced ham an' vegetables.
4. Pour mixture evenly into the muffin tin.
5. Bake for 20 25 minutes until set an' lightly golden.
6. Allow to cool slightly before servin'.

Nutritional data (approximate) for each servin':
- Calories: 120
- Protein: 10g
- Carbohydrates: 2g
- Fat: 8g

Suggestions for freezin' an' storage:
- Store egg muffins in an airtight container in the refrigerator for up to 4 days or freeze individually wrapped for up to 3 months. Reheat in the microwave.

Reasons why this recipe stands out:
- Provides a convenient an' customizable breakfast option that's high in protein an' packed with vegetables for added nutrition.

Poached Eggs on Whole Wheat Toast with Avocado

Prep Time: 15 minutes

Ingredients:

- 2 eggs
- 2 slices whole wheat toast
- 1/2 avocado, sliced
- Salt an' pepper to taste

Step by step instructions:
1. Brin' a pot of water to a gentle simmer.
2. Crack eggs into individual small bowls or cups.
3. Carefully slide eggs into the simmerin' water an' cook for 3 4 minutes for a soft yolk.
4. While eggs are cookin', toast the whole wheat bread slices.
5. Remove eggs with a slotted spoon an' drain excess water.
6. Place poached eggs on top of toasted bread slices.
7. Top with sliced avocado an' season with salt an' pepper.

Nutritional data (approximate) for each servin':
- Calories: 300
- Protein: 15g
- Carbohydrates: 24g
- Fat: 16g

Suggestions for freezin' an' storage:
- This dish is best enjoyed fresh an' not suitable for freezin'. Store any leftovers in the refrigerator for up to 2 days.

Reasons why this recipe stands out:
- Offers a simple yet satisfyin' breakfast option featurin' creamy avocado an' perfectly poached eggs on whole wheat toast, providin' a balanced mix of protein, healthy fats, an' carbohydrates.

Smoothies with Protein Powder, Greens, an' Low Sugar Fruits (like mango)

Prep Time: 5 minutes

Ingredients:

- 1 cup frozen mango chunks
- Handful of spinach or kale
- 1 scoop protein powder (flavor of your choice)
- 1/2 cup water or unsweetened almond milk

Step by step instructions:
1. Combine all ingredients in a blender.
2. Blend until smooth an' creamy.
3. Add more liquid if needed to reach desired consistency.
4. Pour into a glass an' enjoy immediately.

Nutritional data (approximate) for each servin':
- Calories: 250
- Protein: 20g
- Carbohydrates: 30g
- Fat: 5g

Suggestions for freezin' an' storage:
- Smoothies are best enjoyed fresh but can be stored in the refrigerator for up to 24 hours.

Reasons why this recipe stands out:
- Incorporates protein powder for an added protein boost, along with nutrient rich greens an' low sugar fruits like mango, creatin' a refreshin' an' nourishin' breakfast option.

Greek Yogurt Parfait with Berries an' a sprinkle of Granola

Prep Time: 5 minutes

Ingredients:

- 1/2 cup Greek yogurt
- Mixed berries (strawberries, blueberries, raspberries)
- Granola

Step by step instructions:
1. In a glass or bowl, layer Greek yogurt, mixed berries, an' granola.
2. Repeat layers as desired.
3. Serve immediately.

Nutritional data (approximate) for each servin':
- Calories: 200
- Protein: 15g
- Carbohydrates: 25g
- Fat: 5g

Suggestions for freezin' an' storage:
- Parfaits are best enjoyed fresh but can be stored in the refrigerator for up to 24 hours.

Reasons why this recipe stands out:
- Offers a satisfyin' an' customizable breakfast option with creamy Greek yogurt, fresh berries, an' crunchy granola, providin' a balance of protein, carbohydrates, an' healthy fats.

Breakfast Burrito Bowl with Scrambled Eggs, Black Beans, an' Salsa

Prep Time: 20 minutes

Ingredients:
- 4 eggs
- 1 cup cooked black beans
- 1/2 cup salsa
- 1 avocado, diced
- 1/4 cup chopped cilantro (optional)
- Salt an' pepper to taste

Step by step instructions:
1. Scramble eggs in a skillet over medium heat until cooked through. Season with salt an' pepper.
2. Divide scrambled eggs, black beans, salsa, diced avocado, an' chopped cilantro (if usin') among servin' bowls.
3. Serve hot an' enjoy!

Nutritional data (approximate) for each servin':
- Calories: 320
- Protein: 18g
- Carbohydrates: 30g
- Fat: 15g

Suggestions for freezin' an' storage:
- Store any leftovers in separate airtight containers in the refrigerator for up to 2 days. Reheat gently an' assemble before servin'.

Reasons why this recipe stands out:
- Combines protein rich scrambled eggs an' black beans with flavorful salsa an' creamy avocado for a satisfyin' breakfast bowl packed with nutrients an' flavor.

Lunch & Dinner

Cream of Broccoli Soup (omit heavy cream, use low fat milk)

Prep Time: 25 minutes

Ingredients:

- 1 tablespoon olive oil
- 1 onion, chopped
- 2 cloves garlic, minced
- 4 cups broccoli florets
- 4 cups low sodium vegetable broth
- 1 cup low fat milk

Step by step instructions:
1. Warm olive oil in a saucepan at a medium temperature. Add onion an' garlic, sauté until softened.
2. Add broccoli florets an' vegetable broth. Brin' to a boil, then reduce heat an' simmer until broccoli is tender.
3. Use an immersion blender to blend the soup until smooth.
4. Stir in low fat milk an' heat through.
5. Season with salt an' pepper to taste, then serve hot.

Nutritional data (approximate) for each servin':
- Calories: 150
- Protein: 6g
- Carbohydrates: 20g
- Fat: 5g

Suggestions for freezin' an' storage:
- Cool soup completely before transferrin' to freezer safe containers. Freeze for up to 3 months. Thaw overnight in the refrigerator an' reheat gently on the stove.

Reasons why this recipe stands out:
- Offers a creamy texture without heavy cream, makin' it a healthier option without compromisin' on taste.

Stir-fried Chicken an' Veggies with Brown Rice

Prep Time: 20 minutes

Ingredients:

- 2 chicken breasts, sliced
- 2 cups mixed vegetables (bell peppers, broccoli, carrots)
- 2 tablespoons soy sauce
- 1 tablespoon sesame oil
- 2 cups cooked brown rice

Step by step instructions:

1. Heat sesame oil in a large skillet or wok over medium high heat.
2. Add sliced chicken breasts an' cook until browned an' cooked through.
3. Add mixed vegetables to the skillet an' stir fry until tender crisp.
4. Pour soy sauce over the chicken an' vegetables, stirrin' to combine.
5. Serve hot over cooked brown rice.

Nutritional data (approximate) for each servin':

- Calories: 350
- Protein: 30g
- Carbohydrates: 40g
- Fat: 8g

Suggestions for freezin' an' storage:

- Store leftovers in an airtight container in the refrigerator for up to 3 days. Reheat in the microwave or on the stove.

Reasons why this recipe stands out:

- Provides a balanced meal with lean protein, plenty of vegetables, an' whole grains, all cooked together for a quick an' flavorful dinner.

Salmon with Roasted Asparagus an' Lemon

Prep Time: 25 minutes

Ingredients:

- 4 salmon fillets
- 1 bunch asparagus, trimmed
- 2 tablespoons olive oil
- Salt an' pepper to taste
- Lemon wedges for servin'

Step by step instructions:

1. Preheat oven to 400°F (200°C).
2. Place salmon fillets an' trimmed asparagus on a bakin' sheet.
3. Drizzle with olive oil an' season with salt an' pepper.
4. Roast in the preheated oven for 12 15 minutes, or until salmon is cooked through an' asparagus is tender.
5. Serve hot with lemon wedges.

Nutritional data (approximate) for each servin':
- Calories: 300
- Protein: 25g
- Carbohydrates: 5g
- Fat: 20g

Suggestions for freezin' an' storage:
- Store any leftovers in an airtight container in the refrigerator for up to 2 days. Reheat gently in the microwave or enjoy cold in salads or wraps.

Reasons why this recipe stands out:
- Offers a simple yet elegant dish packed with omega 3 fatty acids from salmon an' nutritious asparagus, perfect for a healthy dinner option.

Turkey Burgers on Whole Wheat Buns with Sweet Potato Fries

Prep Time: 30 minutes

Ingredients:

- 1 lb ground turkey
- 1/4 cup breadcrumbs
- 1 egg
- 1 teaspoon garlic powder
- 1 teaspoon onion powder
- Salt an' pepper to taste
- Whole wheat burger buns
- Sweet potatoes, cut into fries

Step by step instructions:

1. In a bowl, mix together ground turkey, breadcrumbs, egg, garlic powder, onion powder, salt, an' pepper.
2. Form the mixture into burger patties.
3. Cook turkey burgers on a grill or skillet over medium heat until cooked through, about 6 - 8 minutes per side.
4. Meanwhile, bake sweet potato fries in the oven accordin' to package instructions.
5. Serve turkey burgers on whole wheat buns with sweet potato fries on the side.

Nutritional data (approximate) for each servin':
- Calories: 400
- Protein: 30g
- Carbohydrates: 35g
- Fat: 15g

Suggestions for freezin' an' storage:
- Freeze uncooked burger patties individually on a bakin' sheet, then transfer to a freezer bag for up to 3 months. Cook from frozen, addin' a few extra minutes to the cookin' time.

Reasons why this recipe stands out:
- Provides a leaner alternative to beef burgers with the added benefit of sweet potato fries for a satisfyin' an' wholesome meal.

Lentil Soup with Whole Wheat Bread

Prep Time: 40 minutes

Ingredients:

- 1 cup dried lentils
- 1 onion, chopped
- 2 carrots, diced
- 2 stalks celery, diced
- 2 cloves garlic, minced
- 4 cups vegetable broth
- 1 can diced tomatoes
- 1 teaspoon dried thyme
- Salt an' pepper to taste
- Whole wheat bread for servin'

Step by step instructions:
1. Rinse lentils under cold water an' drain.
2. In a large pot, heat olive oil over medium heat. Add onion, carrots, celery, an' garlic. Cook until vegetables are softened.
3. Add lentils, vegetable broth, diced tomatoes, an' dried thyme to the pot. Brin' to a boil, then reduce heat an' simmer for 25 30 minutes, or until lentils are tender.
4. Season with salt an' pepper to taste.
5. Serve hot with whole wheat bread.

Nutritional data (approximate) for each servin':
- Calories: 250
- Protein: 15g
- Carbohydrates: 45g
- Fat: 2g

Suggestions for freezin' an' storage:
- Cool soup completely before transferrin' to freezer safe containers. Freeze for up to 3 months. Thaw overnight in the refrigerator an' reheat gently on the stove.

Reasons why this recipe stands out:
- Offers a hearty an' nutritious soup packed with protein an' fiber from lentils, perfect for a comfortin' meal on chilly days.

Baked Cod with Roasted Tomatoes an' Herbs

Prep Time: 30 minutes

Ingredients:
- 4 cod fillets
- 2 cups cherry tomatoes
- 2 tablespoons olive oil
- 2 cloves garlic, minced
- 1 teaspoon dried basil
- 1 teaspoon dried oregano
- Salt an' pepper to taste

Step by step instructions:
1. Preheat oven to 400°F (200°C).
2. Place cod fillets in a bakin' dish.
3. In a bowl, toss cherry tomatoes with olive oil, minced garlic, dried basil, dried oregano, salt, an' pepper.
4. Arrange tomatoes around the cod fillets in the bakin' dish.
5. Bake in the preheated oven for 15 20 minutes, or until fish is cooked through an' tomatoes are softened.

Nutritional data (approximate) for each servin':
- Calories: 200
- Protein: 25g
- Carbohydrates: 5g
- Fat: 8g

Suggestions for freezin' an' storage:
- Store any leftovers in an airtight container in the refrigerator for up to 2 days. Reheat gently in the microwave or enjoy cold in salads or wraps.

Reasons why this recipe stands out:
- Delivers a light an' flavorful dish featurin' flaky cod paired with juicy roasted tomatoes an' aromatic herbs, offerin' a simple yet elegant dinner option.

<u>Chicken Noodle Soup (use thin noodles an' low sodium broth)</u>

Prep Time: 35 minutes

Ingredients:
- 2 chicken breasts, cooked an' shredded
- 6 cups low sodium chicken broth
- 2 carrots, sliced
- 2 celery stalks, sliced
- 1 onion, chopped
- 2 cloves garlic, minced
- 2 cups thin egg noodles
- Salt an' pepper to taste

Step by step instructions:
1. In a large pot, brin' chicken broth to a boil over medium high heat.
2. Add carrots, celery, onion, an' garlic to the pot. Reduce heat an' simmer until vegetables are tender.
3. Stir in shredded chicken an' thin egg noodles. Cook until noodles are al dente.
4. Season with salt an' pepper to taste.
5. Serve hot.

Nutritional data (approximate) for each servin':
- Calories: 250
- Protein: 20g
- Carbohydrates: 25g
- Fat: 8g

Suggestions for freezin' an' storage:
- Cool soup completely before transferrin' to freezer safe containers. Freeze for up to 3 months. Thaw overnight in the refrigerator an' reheat gently on the stove.

Reasons why this recipe stands out:
- Offers a comfortin' an' classic soup with the goodness of chicken, vegetables, an' noodles, perfect for warmin' up on chilly evenings.

Poached Chicken Breast with Quinoa an' Roasted Vegetables

Prep Time: 40 minutes

Ingredients:
- 2 chicken breasts
- 1 cup quinoa
- 2 cups mixed vegetables (bell peppers, zucchini, cherry tomatoes)
- 2 tablespoons olive oil
- Salt an' pepper to taste

Step by step instructions:
1. Poach chicken breasts in simmerin' water until cooked through, about 15 20 minutes. Remove from water an' let cool before slicin'.
2. Cook quinoa accordin' to package instructions.
3. Preheat oven to 400°F (200°C).
4. Toss mixed vegetables with olive oil, salt, an' pepper. Spread on a bakin' sheet.
5. Roast vegetables in the preheated oven for 20 25 minutes, or until tender an' lightly browned.
6. Serve sliced poached chicken breast with cooked quinoa an' roasted vegetables.

Nutritional data (approximate) for each servin':
- Calories: 400
- Protein: 30g
- Carbohydrates: 35g
- Fat: 15g

Suggestions for freezin' an' storage:
- Store any leftovers in separate airtight containers in the refrigerator for up to 3 days. Reheat gently in the microwave or on the stove.

Reasons why this recipe stands out:
- Provides a balanced meal with lean protein from chicken, fiber an' nutrients from quinoa, an' a variety of vitamins an' minerals from roasted vegetables, makin' it a wholesome an' satisfyin' dish.

Vegetarian Chili with Kidney Beans an' Corn

Prep Time: 45 minutes

Ingredients:
- 2 tablespoons olive oil
- 1 onion, chopped
- 2 cloves garlic, minced
- 1 bell pepper, diced
- 1 zucchini, diced
- 1 can (15 oz) kidney beans, drained an' rinsed
- 1 can (15 oz) corn kernels, drained
- 1 can (15 oz) diced tomatoes
- 2 cups vegetable broth
- 2 teaspoons chili powder
- 1 teaspoon cumin
- Salt an' pepper to taste

Step by step instructions:

1. In a large pot, warm olive oil over medium heat. Add onion an' garlic, sauté until softened.
2. Add bell pepper an' zucchini, cook until vegetables are tender.
3. Stir in kidney beans, corn, diced tomatoes, vegetable broth, chili powder, an' cumin.
4. Brin' to a boil, then reduce heat an' simmer for 25 - 30 minutes, stirrin' occasionally.
5. Season with salt an' pepper to taste.
6. Serve hot.

Nutritional data (approximate) for each servin':
- Calories: 250
- Protein: 10g
- Carbohydrates: 40g
- Fat: 6g

Suggestions for freezin' an' storage:

- Cool chili completely before transferrin' to freezer safe containers. Freeze for up to 3 months. Thaw overnight in the refrigerator an' reheat gently on the stove.

Reasons why this recipe stands out:

- Offers a hearty an' flavorful chili packed with protein an' fiber from kidney beans an' corn, makin' it a satisfyin' an' nutritious meal option for vegetarians.

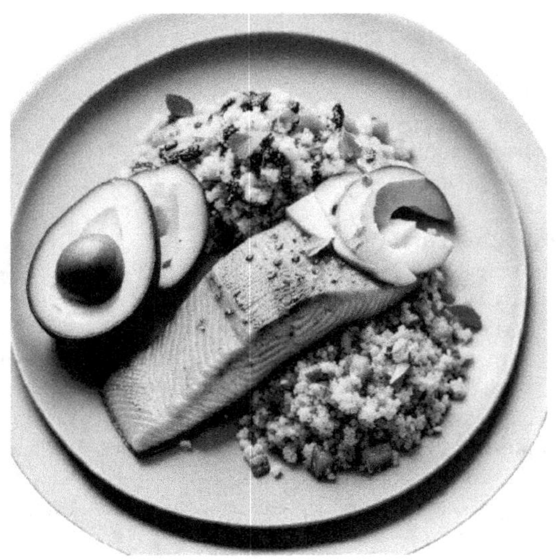

Turkey Meatloaf with Mashed Cauliflower (use low fat milk)

Prep Time: 1 hour

Ingredients:

- 1 lb ground turkey
- 1/2 cup breadcrumbs
- 1 onion, finely chopped
- 2 cloves garlic, minced
- 1 egg
- 1/4 cup ketchup
- Salt an' pepper to taste
- 1 head cauliflower, chopped
- 1/4 cup low fat milk

Step by step instructions:

1. Preheat oven to 375°F (190°C).
2. In a bowl, mix together ground turkey, breadcrumbs, onion, garlic, egg, ketchup, salt, an' pepper.
3. Form the mixture into a loaf an' place in a greased loaf pan.
4. Bake in the preheated oven for 45 50 minutes, or until cooked through.
5. Meanwhile, steam cauliflower until tender. Drain an' mash with low fat milk until smooth.
6. Serve slices of turkey meatloaf with mashed cauliflower on the side.

Nutritional data (approximate) for each servin':

- Calories: 300
- Protein: 25g
- Carbohydrates: 20g
- Fat: 12g

Suggestions for freezin' an' storage:

- Freeze any leftovers in an airtight container for up to 3 months. Thaw overnight in the refrigerator an' reheat gently in the microwave or oven.

Reasons why this recipe stands out:

- Presents a healthier version of classic meatloaf usin' lean ground turkey, paired with creamy mashed cauliflower for a nutritious twist on a comfort food favorite.

Vegetarian Chili with Kidney Beans an' Cornbread

Prep Time: 20 minutes

Ingredients:
- 1 can (15 oz) kidney beans, drained an' rinsed
- 1 can (15 oz) diced tomatoes
- 1 onion, diced
- 1 bell pepper, diced
- 2 cloves garlic, minced
- 1 tablespoon chili powder
- 1 teaspoon cumin
- Salt an' pepper to taste

Step by step instructions:
- In a large pot, sauté onion, bell pepper, an' garlic until softened.
- Add diced tomatoes, kidney beans, chili powder, cumin, salt, an' pepper.
- Brin' to a simmer an' cook for 15 20 minutes.
- Serve hot with cornbread

Nutritional data (approximate) for each servin':
- Calories: 250
- Protein: 10g
- Carbohydrates: 45g
- Fat: 2g

Suggestions for freezin' an' storage:
- Allow chili to cool completely before transferrin' to freezer safe containers. Freeze for up to 3 months. Heat in the microwave or on the stove.

Reasons why this recipe stands out:
- A hearty an' satisfyin' vegetarian meal packed with protein an' fiber, perfect for chilly nights.

One Pan Shrimp an' Asparagus with Lemon Garlic Butter

Prep Time: 15 minutes

Ingredients:

- 1 lb shrimp, peeled an' deveined
- 1 lb asparagus, trimmed
- 3 cloves garlic, minced
- 2 tablespoons butter
- Juice of 1 lemon
- Salt an' pepper to taste

Step by step instructions:
1. Preheat oven to 400°F (200°C).
2. Place shrimp an' asparagus on a bakin' sheet.
3. In a small saucepan, melt butter an' add garlic, lemon juice, salt, an' pepper.
4. Pour the butter mixture over the shrimp an' asparagus.
5. Bake for 10 - 12 minutes until shrimp is pink an' asparagus is tender.

Nutritional data (approximate) for each servin':
- Calories: 200
- Protein: 25g
- Carbohydrates: 8g
- Fat: 8g

Suggestions for freezin' an' storage:
- This dish is best enjoyed fresh but can be stored in an airtight container in the refrigerator for up to 2 days.

Reasons why this recipe stands out:
- Quick an' easy to make, this flavorful dish requires minimal cleanup, makin' it perfect for busy weeknights.

Chicken an' Vegetable Curry with Brown Rice

Prep Time: 25 minutes

Ingredients:

- 1 lb chicken breast, cubed
- 2 cups mixed vegetables (such as bell peppers, carrots, an' peas)
- 1 onion, diced
- 2 cloves garlic, minced
- 1 can (13.5 oz) coconut milk
- 2 tablespoons curry powder
- Salt an' pepper to taste
- Cooked brown rice for servin'

Step by step instructions:

1. In a large skillet, cook chicken until browned on all sides. Remove from skillet an' set aside.
2. In the same skillet, sauté onion an' garlic until softened.
3. Add mixed vegetables an' cook until tender.
4. Return chicken to the skillet an' stir in coconut milk an' curry powder. Season with salt an' pepper.
5. Simmer for 10 - 15 minutes until the chicken is cooked through an' the sauce has thickened.
6. Serve hot over cooked brown rice.

Nutritional data (approximate) for each servin':

- Calories: 400
- Protein: 30g
- Carbohydrates: 20g
- Fat: 20g

Suggestions for freezin' an' storage:

- Allow curry to cool completely before transferrin' to freezer safe containers. Freeze for up to 3 months. Heat in the microwave or on the stove.

Reasons why this recipe stands out:

- A flavorful an' nutritious curry packed with protein an' veggies, perfect for a satisfyin' meal any day of the week.

Turkey Meatballs with Marinara Sauce an' Zucchini Noodles

Prep Time: 30 minutes

Ingredients:

- 1 lb ground turkey
- 1/4 cup breadcrumbs
- 1 egg
- 1 teaspoon Italian seasonin'
- 2 cups marinara sauce
- 4 medium zucchinis, spiralized into noodles

Step by step instructions:
1. Preheat oven to 400°F (200°C).
2. In a bowl, combine ground turkey, breadcrumbs, egg, an' Italian seasonin'. Roll into meatballs.
3. Place meatballs on a bakin' sheet lined with parchment paper an' bake for 15 20 minutes until cooked through.
4. In a skillet, heat marinara sauce until warmed.
5. Add zucchini noodles to the skillet an' cook until tender.
6. Serve meatballs over zucchini noodles with marinara sauce.

Nutritional data (approximate) for each servin':
- Calories: 300
- Protein: 25g
- Carbohydrates: 15g
- Fat: 15g

Suggestions for freezin' an' storage:
- Freeze cooked meatballs separately from the sauce an' zucchini noodles. Reheat in the oven or microwave before servin'.

Reasons why this recipe stands out:
- A healthier twist on a classic favorite, this dish is low carb an' high protein, makin' it a guilt free option for dinner.

Beef Stew with Sweet Potatoes an' Green Beans

Prep Time: 30 minutes

Ingredients:
- 1 lb beef stew meat, cubed
- 2 sweet potatoes, peeled an' cubed
- 1 onion, diced
- 2 cloves garlic, minced
- 2 cups green beans, trimmed
- 4 cups beef broth
- 1 tablespoon tomato paste
- 1 teaspoon thyme
- Salt an' pepper to taste

Step by step instructions:
1. In a large pot, brown beef stew meat over medium heat. Remove from pot an' set aside.
2. In the same pot, sauté onion an' garlic until softened.
3. Add sweet potatoes, green beans, beef broth, tomato paste, thyme, salt, an' pepper.
4. Return beef stew meat to the pot an' brin' to a simmer.
5. Cook for 25 - 30 minutes until the beef is tender an' the vegetables are cooked through.
6. Serve hot.

Nutritional data (approximate) for each servin':
- Calories: 350
- Protein: 25g
- Carbohydrates: 30g
- Fat: 15g

Suggestions for freezin' an' storage:
- Allow stew to cool completely before transferrin' to freezer safe containers. Freeze for up to 3 months. Heat in the microwave or on the stove.

Reasons why this recipe stands out:
- A comfortin' an' hearty stew packed with tender beef an' nutritious vegetables, perfect for a cozy dinner.

Baked Tofu with Peanut Sauce an' Rainbow Vegetables

Prep Time: 35 minutes

Ingredients:

- 1 block tofu, pressed an' cubed
- 2 tablespoons soy sauce
- 1 tablespoon sesame oil
- 1/4 cup peanut butter
- 2 tablespoons rice vinegar
- 1 tablespoon honey or maple syrup
- 2 cups mixed vegetables (such as bell peppers, carrots, an' broccoli)

Step by step instructions:
1. Preheat oven to 400°F (200°C).
2. In a bowl, whisk together soy sauce, sesame oil, peanut butter, rice vinegar, an' honey.
3. Toss tofu cubes in the peanut sauce until well coated.
4. Place tofu on a bakin' sheet lined with parchment paper an' bake for 25 30 minutes until golden an' crispy.
5. In the meantime, steam or stir fry mixed vegetables until tender.
6. Serve baked tofu with rainbow vegetables.

Nutritional data (approximate) for each servin':
- Calories: 300
- Protein: 20g
- Carbohydrates: 20g
- Fat: 15g

Suggestions for freezin' an' storage:
- Store leftover tofu an' vegetables separately in airtight containers in the refrigerator for up to 3 days. Reheat before servin'.

Reasons why this recipe stands out:
- A flavorful an' colorful dish that's packed with plant based protein an' nutrients, makin' it a satisfyin' meatless option for any day of the week.

Lentil Soup with Whole Wheat Bread

Prep Time: 40 minutes

Ingredients:

- 1 cup dried lentils, rinsed an' drained
- 1 onion, diced
- 2 carrots, diced
- 2 stalks celery, diced
- 2 cloves garlic, minced
- 4 cups vegetable broth
- 1 can (14.5 oz) diced tomatoes
- 1 teaspoon dried thyme
- Salt an' pepper to taste

Step by step instructions:
1. In a large pot, sauté onion, carrots, celery, an' garlic until softened.
2. Add lentils, vegetable broth, diced tomatoes, thyme, salt, an' pepper to the pot.
3. Brin' to a boil, then reduce heat an' simmer for 25 30 minutes until lentils are tender.
4. Adjust seasonin' if needed an' serve hot with whole wheat bread.

Nutritional data (approximate) for each servin':
- Calories: 250
- Protein: 15g
- Carbohydrates: 40g
- Fat: 2g

Suggestions for freezin' an' storage:
- Allow soup to cool completely before transferrin' to freezer safe containers. Freeze for up to 3 months. Heat in the microwave or on the stove.

Reasons why this recipe stands out:
- A nutritious an' comfortin' soup that's rich in protein an' fiber, perfect for a satisfyin' meal on a chilly day.

Poached Salmon with Quinoa Salad an' Avocado Dressin'

Prep Time: 30 minutes

Ingredients:
- 4 salmon fillets
- 1 cup quinoa, rinsed
- 2 cups water or vegetable broth
- 1 avocado
- Juice of 1 lime
- 2 tablespoons olive oil
- Salt an' pepper to taste

Step by step instructions:
1. In a pot, brin' water or vegetable broth to a boil. Add quinoa, reduce heat, cover, an' simmer for 15 20 minutes until cooked.
2. In the meantime, prepare the avocado dressin' by blendin' avocado, lime juice, olive oil, salt, an' pepper until smooth.
3. Season salmon fillets with salt an' pepper, then place in a skillet with enough water to cover halfway. Brin' to a simmer an' poach for 8 10 minutes until cooked through.
4. Fluff quinoa with a fork an' serve with poached salmon an' avocado dressin'.

Nutritional data (approximate) for each servin':
- Calories: 400
- Protein: 25g
- Carbohydrates: 30g
- Fat: 20g

Suggestions for freezin' an' storage:
- Store leftover salmon, quinoa, an' avocado dressin' separately in airtight containers in the refrigerator for up to 2 days. Reheat before servin'.

Reasons why this recipe stands out:
- A healthy an' flavorful meal featurin' omega 3 rich salmon, protein packed quinoa, an' a creamy avocado dressin', perfect for a nutritious dinner option.

Black Bean Burgers with Coleslaw on Whole Wheat Buns

Prep Time: 40 minutes

Ingredients:
- 2 cans (15 oz each) black beans, drained an' rinsed
- 1/2 cup breadcrumbs
- 1/4 cup finely chopped onion
- 2 cloves garlic, minced
- 1 teaspoon cumin
- 1 teaspoon chili powder
- Salt an' pepper to taste
- 4 whole wheat burger buns
- Coleslaw mix (cabbage, carrots, etc.)
- Your favorite burger toppings (lettuce, tomato, onion, etc.)

Step by step instructions:
1. In a large bowl, mash black beans with a fork or potato masher until mostly smooth.
2. Add breadcrumbs, onion, garlic, cumin, chili powder, salt, an' pepper to the mashed beans. Mix until well combined.
3. Divide the mixture into 4 equal portions an' shape each portion into a burger patty.
4. Heat a skillet over medium heat an' lightly oil the surface.
5. Cook the black bean burgers for 4 5 minutes on each side, or until heated through an' golden brown.
6. Toast whole wheat burger buns if desired, then assemble burgers with coleslaw an' your favorite toppings.

Nutritional data (approximate) for each servin':
- Calories: 350
- Protein: 15g
- Carbohydrates: 60g
- Fat: 5g

Suggestions for freezin' an' storage:
- Freeze uncooked black bean burger patties individually on a bakin' sheet, then transfer to a freezer bag for up to 3 months. Cook from frozen, addin' a few extra minutes to the cookin' time.

Reasons why this recipe stands out:

- A delicious an' nutritious vegetarian option that's packed with protein an' fiber. The black bean burgers are flavorful an' satisfyin', especially when paired with crunchy coleslaw an' whole wheat buns.

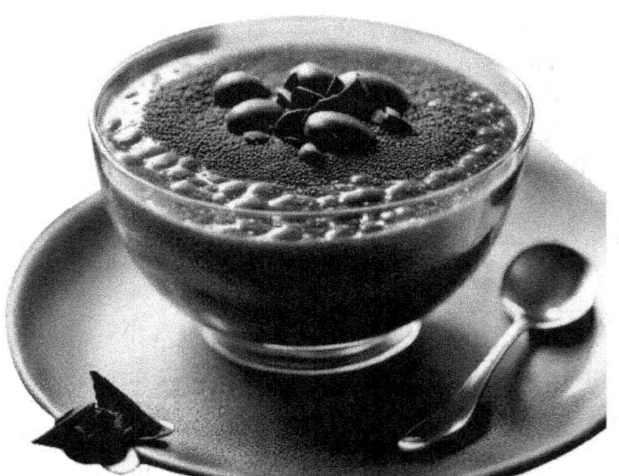

Chicken Fajita Bowls with Cilantro Lime Rice

Prep Time: 30 minutes

Ingredients:
- 1 lb chicken breast, sliced
- 2 bell peppers, thinly sliced
- 1 onion, thinly sliced
- 2 tablespoons fajita seasonin'
- 2 cups cooked rice
- Juice of 2 limes
- 1/4 cup chopped cilantro
- Salt an' pepper to taste
- Optional toppings: salsa, avocado, sour cream, shredded cheese

Step by step instructions:
1. In a bowl, toss sliced chicken breast with fajita seasonin' until evenly coated.
2. Heat a skillet over medium high heat an' add chicken. Cook for 5 6 minutes until browned an' cooked through. Remove from skillet an' set aside.
3. In the same skillet, add sliced bell peppers an' onion. Cook until tender an' slightly charred, about 5 6 minutes.
4. In a separate bowl, mix cooked rice with lime juice, cilantro, salt, an' pepper.
5. Assemble fajita bowls by dividin' the cilantro lime rice among servin' bowls, then toppin' with cooked chicken, bell peppers, an' onion.
6. Serve hot with optional toppings.

Nutritional data (approximate) for each servin':
- Calories: 400
- Protein: 30g
- Carbohydrates: 45g
- Fat: 10g

Suggestions for freezin' an' storage:
- Store leftover components separately in airtight containers in the refrigerator for up to 2 days. Reheat before servin' an' assemble fresh bowls.

Reasons why this recipe stands out:
- These chicken fajita bowls are burstin' with flavor from the seasoned chicken, colorful peppers, an' zesty cilantro lime rice. They're customizable with various toppings an' perfect for a satisfyin' meal.

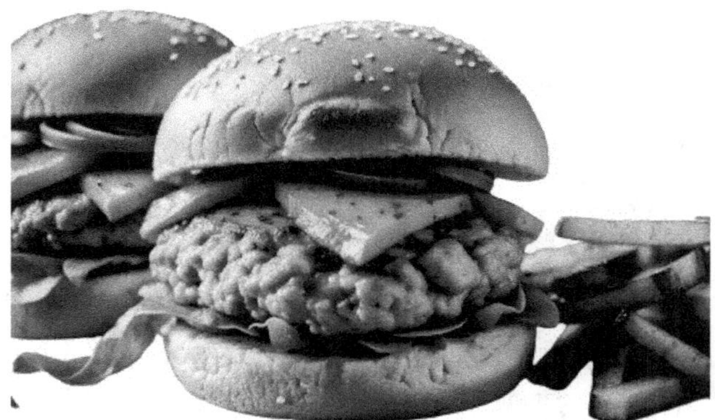

Snacks

Cottage Cheese with Sliced Cucumber an' Dill

Prep Time: 5 minutes

Ingredients:

- 1/2 cup cottage cheese
- 1/2 cucumber, sliced
- Fresh dill, chopped

Step by step instructions:
1. Place cottage cheese in a bowl.
2. Top with sliced cucumber.
3. Sprinkle with fresh dill.
4. Enjoy as a quick an' refreshin' snack.

Nutritional data (approximate) for each servin':
- Calories: 120
- Protein: 12g
- Carbohydrates: 8g
- Fat: 4g

Suggestions for freezin' an' storage:
- Best enjoyed fresh, but leftovers can be stored in an airtight container in the refrigerator for up to 2 days.

Reasons why this recipe stands out:
- Offers a light an' protein rich snack option with the freshness of cucumber an' dill.

Hard boiled Eggs with Celery Sticks

Prep Time: 15 minutes

Ingredients:
- 2 eggs
- Celery sticks

Step by step instructions:
1. Place eggs in a saucepan an' cover with water.
2. Brin' to a boil, then reduce heat an' simmer for 10 minutes.
3. Remove eggs from heat an' run under cold water to cool.
4. Peel eggs an' serve with celery sticks.

Nutritional data (approximate) for each servin':
- Calories: 140
- Protein: 12g
- Carbohydrates: 2g
- Fat: 10g

Suggestions for freezin' an' storage:
- Hard boiled eggs can be stored in the refrigerator for up to 1 week. Keep celery sticks fresh by wrappin' them in damp paper towels an' storin' them in a sealed bag or container.

Reasons why this recipe stands out:
- Provides a protein packed snack with the crunch of celery, perfect for satisfyin' hunger between meals.

Sliced Bell Peppers with Hummus

Prep Time: 10 minutes

Ingredients:
- Bell peppers, sliced
- Hummus

Step by step instructions:
1. Wash an' slice bell peppers.
2. Serve with hummus for dippin'.

Nutritional data (approximate) for each servin':
- Calories: 80
- Protein: 2g
- Carbohydrates: 10g
- Fat: 4g

Suggestions for freezin' an' storage:
- Bell peppers can be stored in the refrigerator for up to 1 week. Store hummus in an airtight container in the refrigerator for up to 1 week.

Reasons why this recipe stands out:
- Offers a colorful an' nutritious snack with the crunch of bell peppers an' the creaminess of hummus.

Apple Slices with Almond Butter

Prep Time: 5 minutes

Ingredients:
- Apple, sliced
- Almond butter

Step by step instructions:
1. Wash an' slice apple.
2. Serve with almond butter for dippin' or spreadin'.

Nutritional data (approximate) for each servin':
- Calories: 150
- Protein: 3g
- Carbohydrates: 20g
- Fat: 8g

Suggestions for freezin' an' storage:
- Apples can be stored in the refrigerator for up to 1 week. Store almond butter in an airtight container in the pantry or refrigerator.

Reasons why this recipe stands out:
- Combines the sweetness of apples with the richness of almond butter for a satisfyin' an' nutritious snack.

Greek Yogurt with Berries an' a sprinkle of Chia Seeds

Prep Time: 5 minutes

Ingredients:
- Greek yogurt
- Mixed berries
- Chia seeds

Step by step instructions:
1. Spoon Greek yogurt into a bowl.
2. Top with mixed berries.
3. Sprinkle with chia seeds.
4. Enjoy as a quick an' nutritious snack or breakfast.

Nutritional data (approximate) for each servin':
- Calories: 180
- Protein: 15g
- Carbohydrates: 20g
- Fat: 5g

Suggestions for freezin' an' storage:
- Greek yogurt can be stored in the refrigerator for up to 2 weeks. Store berries an' chia seeds in airtight containers in the refrigerator.

Reasons why this recipe stands out:
- Provides a protein rich snack with the antioxidant benefits of berries an' the omega 3s from chia seeds.

Carrot Sticks with Low Fat Ranch Dressin'

Prep Time: 10 minutes

Ingredients:
- Carrot sticks
- Low fat ranch dressin'

Step by step instructions:
1. Wash an' peel carrots, then slice into sticks.
2. Serve with low fat ranch dressin' for dippin'.

Nutritional data (approximate) for each servin':
- Calories: 70
- Protein: 2g
- Carbohydrates: 10g
- Fat: 3g

Suggestions for freezin' an' storage:
- Carrot sticks can be stored in the refrigerator for up to 1 week. Store ranch dressin' in an airtight container in the refrigerator.

Reasons why this recipe stands out:
- Offers a crunchy an' satisfyin' snack option with the added flavor of low fat ranch dressin'.

Sugar Free Jello (use unsweetened gelatin an' sugar substitutes)

Prep Time: 5 minutes (plus chillin' time)

Ingredients:
- Unsweetened gelatin
- Sugar substitutes

Step by step instructions:
1. Follow package instructions to prepare sugar free Jello usin' unsweetened gelatin an' sugar substitutes.
2. Pour into molds or a dish an' refrigerate until set.
3. Serve chilled.

Nutritional data (approximate) for each servin':
- Calories: 10
- Protein: 2g
- Carbohydrates: 0g
- Fat: 0g

Suggestions for freezin' an' storage:
- Store sugar free Jello in an airtight container in the refrigerator for up to 1 week.

Reasons why this recipe stands out:
- Provides a low calorie, sugar free alternative to traditional Jello, perfect for those watchin' their sugar intake.

Roasted Chickpeas with Spices (use low sodium options)

Prep Time: 5 minutes (plus bakin' time)

Ingredients:
- Chickpeas (canned or cooked)
- Spices (such as paprika, cumin, garlic powder)

Step by step instructions:
1. Preheat oven to 400°F (200°C).
2. Rinse an' drain chickpeas, then pat dry with a towel.
3. Toss chickpeas with spices of your choice.
4. Spread chickpeas in a single layer on a bakin' sheet lined with parchment paper.
5. Bake for 25 30 minutes or until crispy, shakin' the pan occasionally.
6. Let cool before servin'.

Nutritional data (approximate) for each servin':
- Calories: 150
- Protein: 6g
- Carbohydrates: 25g
- Fat: 2g

Suggestions for freezin' an' storage:
- Store roasted chickpeas in an airtight container at room temperature for up to 1 week.

Reasons why this recipe stands out:
- Offers a crunchy an' flavorful snack option with the added protein an' fiber benefits of chickpeas.

Rice Cakes with Sliced Avocado

Prep Time: 5 minutes

Ingredients:
- Rice cakes
- Avocado, sliced

Step by step instructions:
1. Place rice cakes on a plate.
2. Top each rice cake with sliced avocado.
3. Sprinkle with a pinch of salt an' pepper, if desired.
4. Enjoy as a quick an' satisfyin' snack.

Nutritional data (approximate) for each servin':
- Calories: 120
- Protein: 2g
- Carbohydrates: 15g
- Fat: 6g

Suggestions for freezin' an' storage:
- Rice cakes can be stored in an airtight container in the pantry for several months. Store leftover avocado in an airtight container in the refrigerator with a squeeze of lemon juice to prevent brownin'.

Reasons why this recipe stands out:
- Combines the crispiness of rice cakes with the creaminess of avocado for a satisfyin' an' nutritious snack.

Edamame Pods with a sprinkle of Sea Salt

Prep Time: 5 minutes (if usin' frozen edamame)

Ingredients:
- Edamame pods (fresh or frozen)
- Sea salt

Step by step instructions:
1. If usin' frozen edamame, thaw accordin' to package instructions.
2. Steam edamame pods until tender, about 5 minutes.
3. Sprinkle with sea salt.
4. Enjoy warm or chilled as a nutritious snack.

Nutritional data (approximate) for each servin':
- Calories: 100
- Protein: 9g
- Carbohydrates: 8g
- Fat: 4g

Suggestions for freezin' an' storage:
- Store cooked edamame pods in an airtight container in the refrigerator for up to 3 days.

Reasons why this recipe stands out:
- Provides a protein rich snack with the natural sweetness of edamame an' the added flavor of sea salt.

Drinks

Herbal Tea (variety of flavors)

Prep Time: 5 minutes

Ingredients:
- Herbal tea bags (variety of flavors)
- Hot water

Step by step instructions:
1. Boil water in a kettle.
2. Place herbal tea bag in a cup.
3. Pour hot water over the tea bag.
4. Steep accordin' to package instructions.
5. Remove tea bag an' enjoy.

Nutritional data (approximate) for each servin':
- Calories: 0
- Protein: 0g
- Carbohydrates: 0g
- Fat: 0g

Suggestions for freezin' an' storage:
- Herbal tea bags can be stored in a cool, dry place for an extended period.

Reasons why this recipe stands out:
- Provides a soothin' an' flavorful beverage option without any added calories or caffeine.

Water with Lemon or Cucumber Slices

Prep Time: 5 minutes

Ingredients:
- Water
- Lemon or cucumber slices

Step by step instructions:
1. Fill a pitcher or glass with water.
2. Add lemon or cucumber slices.
3. Stir gently.
4. Let it sit for a few minutes to infuse.
5. Serve chilled or over ice.

Nutritional data (approximate) for each servin':
- Calories: 0
- Protein: 0g
- Carbohydrates: 0g
- Fat: 0g

Suggestions for freezin' an' storage:
- Best served fresh, but leftover infused water can be stored in the refrigerator for up to 24 hours.

Reasons why this recipe stands out:
- Refreshin' an' hydratin', this infused water adds a hint of flavor without any added sugars or calories.

Unsweetened Almond Milk

Prep Time: 5 minutes (if homemade)

Ingredients:
- Almonds (if makin' homemade)
- Water (if makin' homemade)

Step by step instructions (for homemade almond milk):
1. Soak almonds in water overnight.
2. Rinse almonds an' blend with fresh water until smooth.
3. Strain through a nut milk bag or fine sieve.
4. Store in airtight container in the refrigerator.
5. Shake well before usin'.

Nutritional data (approximate) for each servin':
- Calories: 30 - 40 (varies dependin' on brand)
- Protein: 1g
- Carbohydrates: 1g
- Fat: 3g

Suggestions for freezin' an' storage:
- Store in the refrigerator an' consume within 5 7 days.

Reasons why this recipe stands out:
- A dairy free alternative rich in vitamins an' minerals, perfect for those with lactose intolerance or dairy allergies.

Low Sugar Electrolyte Drinks (check labels for sugar content)

Prep Time: Varies (dependin' on if homemade or store bought)

Ingredients:

- Electrolyte drink mix or ingredients for homemade version

Step by step instructions (for homemade version):
1. Mix water with a pinch of salt an' a splash of citrus juice (such as lemon or lime).
2. Optionally, add a small amount of natural sweetener like honey or stevia, if desired.
3. Stir well until everythin' is dissolved.
4. Taste an' adjust as needed.
5. Serve chilled or over ice.

Nutritional data (approximate) for each servin' (varies dependin' on ingredients):
- Calories: Varies
- Protein: 0g
- Carbohydrates: Varies
- Fat: 0g

Suggestions for freezin' an' storage:
- Store homemade electrolyte drinks in the refrigerator for up to 3 days. Store bought drinks follow the manufacturer's instructions.

Reasons why this recipe stands out:
- Offers hydration an' electrolyte replenishment with minimal added sugars, perfect for post workout recovery or stayin' hydrated throughout the day.

Decaf Coffee with Unsweetened Nut Milk

Prep Time: 5 minutes

Ingredients:
- Decaf coffee
- Unsweetened nut milk (such as almond or cashew milk)

Step by step instructions:
1. Brew decaf coffee usin' your preferred method.
2. Heat nut milk in a saucepan or microwave until warm.
3. Pour decaf coffee into a mug.
4. Add warmed nut milk to the coffee.
5. Stir well an' enjoy.

Nutritional data (approximate) for each servin':
- Calories: 10 - 20 (varies dependin' on nut milk)
- Protein: 0g
- Carbohydrates: 1 - 2g (varies dependin' on nut milk)
- Fat: 1 - 2g (varies dependin' on nut milk)

Suggestions for freezin' an' storage:
- Store leftover coffee an' nut milk separately in the refrigerator for up to 2 days. Reheat gently before servin'.

Reasons why this recipe stands out:
- Provides a comfortin' an' caffeine free alternative to regular coffee, with the creamy richness of unsweetened nut milk.

<u>Vegetable Juice (low sodium options)</u>

Prep Time: 10 minutes

Ingredients:
- Assorted vegetables (such as carrots, celery, tomatoes, spinach)
- Optional: lemon or lime juice, herbs (like parsley or cilantro)

Step by step instructions:
1. Wash an' chop vegetables into manageable pieces.
2. Juice the vegetables usin' a juicer or blender.
3. If usin' a blender, strain the juice through a fine mesh sieve or nut milk bag to remove pulp.
4. Add lemon or lime juice an' herbs for extra flavor, if desired.
5. Serve immediately over ice.

Nutritional data (approximate) for each servin':
- Calories: 50 - 100 (varies dependin' on vegetables used)
- Protein: 2 - 4g (varies dependin' on vegetables used)
- Carbohydrates: 10 - 20g (varies dependin' on vegetables used)
- Fat: 0 - 1g (varies dependin' on vegetables used)

Suggestions for freezin' an' storage:
- Best consumed fresh for optimal nutrient content. Store any leftovers in an airtight container in the refrigerator for up to 24 hours.

Reasons why this recipe stands out:
- Provides a nutritious an' low calorie option for gettin' your daily dose of vegetables, ideal for those lookin' to increase their veggie intake.

Clear Broth

Prep Time: 10 minutes

Ingredients:
- Chicken, beef, or vegetable broth

Step by step instructions:
1. Heat the broth in a saucepan over medium heat until warmed through.
2. Optionally, season with a pinch of salt an' pepper to taste.
3. Serve hot in a mug or bowl.
4. Garnish with fresh herbs, if desired.
5. Enjoy as is or use it as a base for soups or stews.

Nutritional data (approximate) for each servin':
- Calories: 10 - 20 (varies dependin' on type of broth)
- Protein: 1 - 2g (varies dependin' on type of broth)
- Carbohydrates: 1 - 2g (varies dependin' on type of broth)
- Fat: 0 - 1g (varies dependin' on type of broth)

Suggestions for freezin' an' storage:
- Store any leftover broth in an airtight container in the refrigerator for up to 5 days or freeze for longer storage.

Reasons why this recipe stands out:
- Provides a comfortin' an' warmin' beverage option, especially durin' colder months or when feelin' under the weather.

Sugar Free Flavored Water

Prep Time: 5 minutes

Ingredients:
- Water
- Sugar free flavorin' drops or extracts (e.g., vanilla, fruit flavors)

Step by step instructions:
1. Fill a pitcher or glass with water.
2. Add a few drops of sugar free flavorin' drops or extracts.
3. Stir well until the flavor is evenly distributed.
4. Taste an' adjust the flavor intensity if needed.
5. Serve chilled or over ice.

Nutritional data (approximate) for each servin':
- Calories: 0
- Protein: 0g
- Carbohydrates: 0g
- Fat: 0g

Suggestions for freezin' an' storage:
- Best consumed fresh. Store any leftovers in the refrigerator for up to 24 hours.

Reasons why this recipe stands out:
- Offers a refreshin' an' customizable alternative to plain water, perfect for those lookin' to stay hydrated without added sugars or artificial sweeteners.

Homemade Infused Water with Fruits or Herbs

Prep Time: 5 minutes

Ingredients:
- Water
- Fresh fruits (e.g., berries, citrus slices) or herbs (e.g., mint, basil)

Step by step instructions:
1. Fill a pitcher or glass with water.
2. Add your choice of fresh fruits or herbs.
3. Stir gently to release the flavors.
4. Let it sit in the refrigerator for at least an hour to infuse.
5. Serve chilled or over ice.

Nutritional data (approximate) for each servin':
- Calories: 0
- Protein: 0g
- Carbohydrates: 0g
- Fat: 0g

Suggestions for freezin' an' storage:
- Best served fresh. Consume within 24 hours for optimal flavor.

Reasons why this recipe stands out:
- Provides a refreshin' an' hydratin' beverage option infused with natural flavors from fruits or herbs, makin' hydration more enjoyable.

Non Caffeinated Tea (like chamomile or peppermint)

Prep Time: 5 minutes

Ingredients:
- Non caffeinated tea bags (e.g., chamomile, peppermint)
- Hot water

Step by step instructions:
1. Boil water in a kettle.
2. Place non caffeinated tea bag in a cup.
3. Pour hot water over the tea bag.
4. Steep accordin' to package instructions.
5. Remove tea bag an' enjoy.

Nutritional data (approximate) for each servin':
- Calories: 0
- Protein: 0g
- Carbohydrates: 0g
- Fat: 0g

Suggestions for freezin' an' storage:
- Tea bags can be stored in a cool, dry place for an extended period.

Reasons why this recipe stands out:
- Offers a calmin' an' soothin' beverage option, perfect for windin' down in the evenin' or anytime you want to relax without the stimulation of caffeine.

1st Week Meal Plan

Day 1:

- Breakfast: Scrambled Eggs with Spinach an' Goat Cheese (Choose a small portion of spinach)
- Lunch: Cream of Broccoli Soup (opt for a thinner consistency by addin' more broth) with a side of Whole Wheat Toast
- Snack: Cottage Cheese with Sliced Cucumber an' Dill
- Dinner: Baked Cod with Roasted Tomatoes an' Herbs (omit the skin for easier digestion)
- Drink: Herbal Tea (variety of flavors) an' Water with Lemon Slices

Day 2:

- Breakfast: Chia Seed Puddin' with Nut Butter an' Sliced Strawberries (limit the amount of nut butter)
- Lunch: Chicken an' Vegetable Stir Fry with Brown Rice (choose well cooked, soft vegetables)
- Snack: Apple Slices with Almond Butter (cut the apple into thin slices)
- Dinner: Poached Chicken Breast with Quinoa an' Roasted Vegetables (opt for steamed or very well roasted vegetables)
- Drink: Unsweetened Almond Milk an' Vegetable Juice (low sodium)

Day 3:

- Breakfast: Protein Smoothie with Berries an' Unsweetened Greek Yogurt (use a low powered blender for easier digestion)
- Lunch: Lentil Soup with Whole Wheat Bread (crumble the bread into the soup for a softer consistency)
- Snack: Greek Yogurt with Berries an' a sprinkle of Chia Seeds
- Dinner: Turkey Meatloaf with Mashed Cauliflower (use low fat milk an' mash the cauliflower very well)
- Drink: Decaf Coffee with Unsweetened Nut Milk an' Clear Broth

Day 4:

- Breakfast: Baked Oatmeal with Apples an' Cinnamon (use very ripe apples an' cook the oatmeal until soft)
- Lunch: Salmon with Roasted Asparagus an' Lemon (omit the lemon if it irritates your stomach)
- Snack: Carrot Sticks with Low Fat Ranch Dressin' (cut the carrots into thin sticks)
- Dinner: Vegetarian Chili with Kidney Beans an' Corn (mash some of the beans for easier digestion)
- Drink: Sugar Free Flavored Water an' Homemade Infused Water with Fruits or Herbs

Day 5:

- Breakfast: Cottage Cheese Pancakes with Berries (use sugar free pancake mix an' small pancakes)
- Lunch: Chicken Noodle Soup (use thin noodles an' low sodium broth, mash some of the noodles for softer texture)
- Snack: Hard boiled Eggs with Celery Sticks (cut the celery sticks very thin)
- Dinner: Poached Eggs on Whole Wheat Toast with Avocado (mash the avocado for easier digestion)
- Drink: Herbal Tea (variety of flavors) an' Water with Lemon Slices

Day 6:

- Breakfast: Egg Muffins with Vegetables an' Ham (choose well cooked, chopped vegetables)
- Lunch: Turkey Burgers on Whole Wheat Buns with Sweet Potato Fries (bake or air fry the sweet potato fries for a softer texture)
- Snack: Sliced Bell Peppers with Hummus
- Dinner: Cream of Broccoli Soup (omit heavy cream, use low fat milk) with a side of Rice Cakes with Sliced Avocado (mash the avocado)
- Drink: Unsweetened Almond Milk an' Low Sugar Electrolyte Drink (check labels for sugar content)

Day 7:

- Breakfast: Smoothies with Protein Powder, Greens, an' Low Sugar Fruits (like mango) (use a low powered blender for easier digestion)

- Lunch: Baked Cod with Roasted Tomatoes an' Herbs (omit the skin for easier digestion) with a side of Quinoa (opt for pre cooked quinoa for convenience)
    - Snack: Roasted Chickpeas with Spices (use low sodium options)
- Dinner: Chicken an' Vegetable Stir Fry with Brown Rice (choose well cooked, soft vegetables)
- Drink: Decaf Coffee with Unsweetened Nut Milk an' Clear Broth
    - Snacks: Feel free to distribute the remainin' snacks throughout the week based on your hunger cues.

- Desserts: While these are listed as occasional treats, prioritize sugar free options or very small portions.

2nd Week Meal Plan

Day 1:

- Breakfast: Greek Yogurt Parfait with Berries an' a sprinkle of Granola (choose a small amount of granola, crushed for easier digestion)
- Lunch: Poached Chicken Breast with Quinoa Salad (use well cooked quinoa, chop all ingredients finely)
- Snack: Sugar Free Jello (use unsweetened gelatin an' sugar substitutes)
- Dinner: Vegetarian Chili with Kidney Beans an' Corn (mash some of the beans for a smoother consistency)
- Drink: Herbal Tea (variety of flavors) an' Water with Cucumber Slices

Day 2:

- Breakfast: Smoothie with Protein Powder, Greens, an' Low Sugar Fruits (like berries) (use a low powered blender)
- Lunch: Tuna Salad on Whole Wheat Toast (choose canned tuna packed in water an' finely chop all ingredients)
- Snack: Cottage Cheese with Sliced Apple (cut the apple into thin slices)
- Dinner: Baked Salmon with Roasted Brussels Sprouts (steam or roast the Brussels sprouts until very soft)
- Drink: Unsweetened Almond Milk an' Vegetable Juice (low sodium)

Day 3:

- Breakfast: Scrambled Eggs with Chopped Tomatoes an' Herbs (choose well cooked, chopped tomatoes)
- Lunch: Chicken Noodle Soup (use thin noodles an' low sodium broth, remove some noodles for a thinner consistency)
- Snack: Hard boiled Eggs with Sliced Bell Peppers (cut the bell peppers into thin strips)
- Dinner: Turkey Meatloaf with Mashed Sweet Potato (use low fat milk an' mash the sweet potato very well)
- Drink: Decaf Coffee with Unsweetened Nut Milk an' Clear Broth

Day 4:

- Breakfast: Chia Seed Puddin' with Berries an' a sprinkle of Chia Seeds
- Lunch: Lentil Soup with a side of Rice Cakes (crumble the rice cakes into the soup)
- Snack: Edamame Pods with a sprinkle of Sea Salt
- Dinner: Poached Cod with Roasted Asparagus an' Lemon (omit the lemon if it irritates your stomach)
- Drink: Sugar Free Flavored Water an' Homemade Infused Water with Fruits or Herbs

Day 5:

- Breakfast: Baked Oatmeal with mashed Banana an' Cinnamon (use very ripe bananas an' cook the oatmeal until soft)
- Lunch: Turkey Burger Bowl with Deconstructed Lettuce Wrap (omit the bun, finely chop all burger ingredients)
- Snack: Sliced Carrot Sticks with Hummus
- Dinner: Cream of Broccoli Soup (omit heavy cream, use low fat milk, an' blend until smooth)
- Drink: Herbal Tea (variety of flavors) an' Water with Lemon Slices

Day 6:

- [ ] **Breakfast**: Protein Smoothie with Berries an' Unsweetened Greek Yogurt (use a low powered blender for easier digestion)
- [ ] Lunch: Chicken Caesar Salad (use a light Caesar dressin', chop all ingredients finely)
- [ ] Snack: Roasted Chickpeas with Spices (use low sodium options)
- [ ] Dinner: Baked Egg Muffins with Vegetables (choose well cooked, finely chopped vegetables)
- [ ] Drink: Unsweetened Almond Milk an' Low Sugar Electrolyte Drink (check labels for sugar content)

Day 7:

- Breakfast: Cottage Cheese Pancakes with Berries (use sugar free pancake mix an' small pancakes)
- Lunch: Shrimp Scampi with Zucchini Noodles (ensure the shrimp is cooked through an' cut the zucchini noodles very thin)
- Snack: Greek Yogurt with Berries an' a sprinkle of Chia Seeds
- Dinner: Chicken Stir Fry with Brown Rice Noodles (use pre cooked rice noodles for convenience an' choose well cooked, soft vegetables)
- Drink: Decaf Coffee with Unsweetened Nut Milk an' Clear Broth
- Snacks: Feel free to distribute the remainin' snacks throughout the week based on your hunger cues.

3rd Week Meal Plan

Day 1:

- Breakfast: Greek Yogurt Bowl with Berries, a sprinkle of Granola, an' a drizzle of Honey (opt for a small amount of granola an' honey)

- Lunch: Tuna Salad Pita with Chopped Vegetables (use canned tuna packed in water, finely chop all ingredients, an' serve with a small whole wheat pita)

- Snack: Sliced Cucumber with Feta Cheese an' a drizzle of Olive Oil

- Dinner: Baked Chicken Breast with Lemon Herb Quinoa an' Roasted Vegetables (choose well cooked, bite sized vegetables an' a squeeze of lemon, not the whole lemon)

- Drink: Herbal Tea (variety of flavors) an' Water with Lemon Slices

Day 2:

- Breakfast: Scrambled Eggs with Spinach an' Diced Tomatoes (choose well cooked spinach an' chopped tomatoes)
-
- Lunch: Lentil Soup with a side of Whole Wheat Crackers (crumble the crackers into the soup)

- Snack: Cottage Cheese with Pineapple Chunks (cut the pineapple into small pieces)

- Dinner: Salmon with Roasted Asparagus an' a dollop of Pesto (omit the pesto if it irritates your stomach)

- Drink: Unsweetened Almond Milk an' Vegetable Juice (low sodium)

Day 3:

- Breakfast: Smoothie with Protein Powder, Greens, an' Low Sugar Fruits (like mango) (use a low powered blender)

- Lunch: Turkey an' Veggie Wrap (use a small whole wheat tortilla, finely chop all ingredients)

- Snack: Apple Slices with Almond Butter (cut the apple into thin slices)

- Dinner: Vegetarian Moussaka (use a low fat recipe an' ensure vegetables are well cooked an' soft)

- Drink: Decaf Coffee with Unsweetened Nut Milk an' Clear Broth

Day 4:

- Breakfast: Chia Seed Puddin' with Berries an' a sprinkle of Chia Seeds

- Lunch: Chicken Caesar Salad (use a light Caesar dressin', opt for shredded chicken, an' chop all ingredients finely)

- Snack: Edamame Pods with a sprinkle of Sea Salt

- Dinner: Poached Whitefish with Sauteed Zucchini an' Herbs (ensure the fish is cooked through an' cut the zucchini into thin slices)

- Drink: Sugar Free Flavored Water an' Homemade Infused Water with Fruits or Herbs

Day 5:

- Breakfast: Baked Oatmeal with mashed Banana an' a sprinkle of Cinnamon (use very ripe bananas an' cook the oatmeal until soft)

- Lunch: Black Bean Burgers on a bed of Greens (omit the bun, finely chop all burger ingredients)

- Snack: Sliced Bell Peppers with Hummus

- Dinner: Cream of Butternut Squash Soup (omit heavy cream, use low fat milk, an' blend until smooth)

- Drink: Herbal Tea (variety of flavors) an' Water with Lemon Slices

Day 6:

- Breakfast: Protein Smoothie with Berries an' Unsweetened Greek Yogurt (use a low powered blender for easier digestion)

- Lunch: Chicken Souvlaki Bowl with Deconstructed Pita (marinate chicken in a small amount of yogurt, omit the pita, an' serve with chopped vegetables)

- Snack: Roasted Chickpeas with Spices (use low sodium options)

- Dinner: Baked Egg Muffins with Chopped Vegetables an' crumbled Feta Cheese (choose well cooked, finely chopped vegetables an' a small amount of feta)

- Drink: Unsweetened Almond Milk an' Low Sugar Electrolyte Drink (check labels for sugar content)

Day 7:

- Breakfast: Cottage Cheese Pancakes with Berries (use sugar free pancake mix an' small pancakes)

- Lunch: Shrimp Salad Sandwich on Whole Wheat Toast (use finely chopped shrimp an' a light amount of mayonnaise)

- Snack: Greek Yogurt with Berries an' a sprinkle of Chia Seeds

- Dinner: One Pan Lemon Garlic Chicken with Roasted Vegetables (choose well cooked, bite sized vegetables an' a squeeze of lemon)

- Drink: Decaf Coffee with Unsweetened Nut Milk an' Clear Broth

4th Week Meal Plan

Day 1:

- ☐ **Breakfast**: Protein Pancakes with Berries (use a low carbohydrate pancake mix an' a small servin' of berries)

- ☐ **Lunch:** Chicken Caesar Salad (use a light Caesar dressin', opt for shredded chicken, an' remove croutons)

- ☐ **Snack**: Cottage Cheese with Diced Mango (cut the mango into small pieces)

- ☐ **Dinner**: Baked Salmon with Roasted Asparagus Tips (choose the tender tips of asparagus for easier digestion)

- ☐ **Drink**: Herbal Tea (variety of flavors) an' Water with Lemon Slices

Day 2:

- **Breakfast**: Scrambled Eggs with Smoked Salmon an' Spinach (choose a small amount of well cooked spinach)

- **Lunch**: Turkey an' Vegetable Soup (ensure vegetables are well cooked an' soft, consider removin' some for a thinner consistency)

- **Snack**: Hard boiled Eggs with Celery Sticks (cut the celery sticks very thin)

- **Dinner**: Poached Chicken Breast with Quinoa an' Steamed Broccoli Florets

- **Drink**: Unsweetened Almond Milk an' Vegetable Juice (low sodium)

Day 3:

- **Breakfast**: Smoothie with Protein Powder an' Unsweetened Greek Yogurt (use a low powered blender)

- **Lunch**: Tuna Salad with Lettuce Wraps (use canned tuna packed in water an' finely chop all ingredients)

- **Snack**: Sliced Bell Peppers with Guacamole (made with mashed avocado)

- **Dinner**: Shrimp Scampi with Zucchini Noodles (ensure the shrimp is cooked through an' cut the zucchini noodles very thin)

- **Drink**: Decaf Coffee with Unsweetened Nut Milk an' Clear Broth

Day 4:

- **Breakfast**: Baked Oatmeal with Protein Powder an' a sprinkle of Cinnamon (use very ripe bananas for added sweetness, if tolerated)

- **Lunch**: Chicken Breast Sandwich on Whole Wheat Toast (use a thin slice of toast an' finely chop the chicken)

- **Snack**: Edamame Pods with a sprinkle of Sea Salt

- **Dinner**: Baked Cod with Roasted Cherry Tomatoes an' Herbs (omit the herbs if they irritate your stomach)

- **Drink**: Sugar Free Flavored Water an' Homemade Infused Water with Berries

Day 5:

- **Breakfast**: Chia Seed Puddin' with Berries an' a sprinkle of Chia Seeds (use a low carb milk alternative if desired)

- **Lunch**: Lentil Soup with a side of Peeled Mashed Potatoes (omit the skin for easier digestion)

- **Snack**: Cottage Cheese with Sliced Cucumber an' Dill

- **Dinner**: Turkey Meatloaf with Mashed Cauliflower (use low fat milk an' mash the cauliflower very well)

- **Drink**: Herbal Tea (variety of flavors) an' Water with Cucumber Slices

Day 6:

- **Breakfast**: Protein Smoothie with Berries an' a scoop of Unsweetened Nut Butter (use a low powered blender)

- **Lunch**: Chicken Stir Fry with Brown Rice Noodles (pre cooked for convenience, choose well cooked, soft vegetables)

- **Snack**: Roasted Chickpeas with Spices (use low sodium options)

- **Dinner**: Baked Egg Muffins with Chopped Ham an' Cheese (choose well cooked, finely chopped ingredients)

- **Drink**: Unsweetened Almond Milk an' Low Sugar Electrolyte Drink (check labels for sugar content)

Day 7:

- **Breakfast**: Scrambled Eggs with Diced Tomatoes an' a sprinkle of Shredded Cheese (choose well cooked tomatoes)

- **Lunch**: Leftover Baked Salmon with a side of Quinoa (reheat gently)

- **Snack**: Greek Yogurt with Berries an' a sprinkle of Chia Seeds

- **Dinner**: Poached Chicken Breast with Mashed Sweet Potato (use low fat milk an' mash the sweet potato very well)

- **Drink**: Decaf Coffee with Unsweetened Nut Milk an' Clear Broth

Thank you very Much

We hope Diabetes Gastroparesis Diet Cookbook has been a valuable companion on your journey towards managin' both diabetes an' gastroparesis. We understand the challenges you face, an' we're thrilled if this book has helped you navigate meal plannin' an' navigate both conditions with greater confidence.

We'd love to hear from you!

Share Your Gratitude:

- What aspects of the book resonated most with you?
- Did the meal plans provide helpful inspiration for your dietary needs?
- How has this book impacted your approach to managin' your health?

Leave a Review:

Your honest feedback is invaluable in helpin' others discover **DIABETES GASTROPARESIS DIET COOKBOOK BY DR. ALMA W. THYGESEN**

- Share your thoughts on the book's content, organization, an' design on major online retailers (e.g., Amazon, Barnes & Noble).

- Spread the word! Recommend the book to friends, family, or online communities dealin' with similar health concerns.

Together, we can create a supportive network an' empower each other on the path to well being!

Thank you for readin'!

P.S.

Feel free to share your experiences an' recipe modifications on social media usin' the hashtag **#EmpoweredByEveryBite.**